NATURAL WAYS
TO
LOWER YOUR
CHOLESTEROL

NATURAL WAYS
TO
LOWER YOUR
CHOLESTEROL

SAFE, DRUG-FREE WAYS TO CUT CHOLESTEROL LEVELS UP TO

30 POINTS IN 30 DAYS

NORMAN D. FORD

Galahad Books • New York

Natural Ways to Lower Your Cholesterol is not intended as medical advice. Its intention is solely informational and educational. Please consult a medical or health professional should the need for one be indicated. The information in this book lends itself to self-help. For obvious reasons, the author and publisher cannot take the medical or legal responsibility of having the contents herein considered as a prescription for everyone. Either you, or the physician who examines and treats you, must take the responsibility for the uses made of this book.

First Galahad Books edition published in 1997.

Galahad Books
A division of Budget Book Service, Inc.
386 Park Avenue South
New York, NY 10016

Galahad Books is a registered trademark of Budget Book Service, Inc.

Published by arrangement with Keats Publishing, Inc.

Library of Congress Catalog Card Number: 96-79814

ISBN: 0-88365-978-6

Printed in the United States of America.

ACKNOWLEDGMENTS

Most of the research behind this book was derived from studies conducted at some of America's most distinguished university medical centers and from such leading health advisory agencies as the National Institutes of Health, the American Heart Association, the National Academy of Sciences, and the Public Citizen Health Research Group. I also drew extensively on the work of Kenneth Cooper, M.D., and colleagues at the Institute of Aerobics Research, Dallas; on the Cholesterol-Lowering Atherosclerosis Study (CLAS); the China Health Study; the Coronary Primary Prevention Trial; the Framingham Heart Study; the Leisure Time Physical Activity Study; the Lipid Research Clinic's Mortality Follow-Up Study, the Helsinki Heart Study; the Diet-Heart Study; the Coronary Primary Prevention Trial; the Oslo Diet-Smoking Study; the Multiple Risk Factor Intervention Trial; the analysis by Ralph S. Paffenbarger, Ph.D., of the mortality statistics of the 17,000 Harvard Alumnae; the Lifestyle Heart Trial by Dean Ornish, M.D. and Larry Scherwitz, M.D., Ph.D.; the Physicians' Health Study; the Pritikin Program; and the Seven Countries Study.

Virtually all of these studies support the validity and effectiveness of a multi-disciplinary (holistic) approach to healing, and of the 18 natural ways to lower cholesterol described in this book.

So many sources were consulted in researching this book that it is impractical to acknowledge every one. However, I would like to acknowledge my debt to the research carried out by Scott Grundy, Ph.D., of the University of Texas Southwest Medical School, Dallas; George Blackburn, M.D., Ph.D., of Harvard Medical School; William Connor, Ph.D., and Sonja L. Connor M.S., R.D., of Oregon Health Sciences University, Portland, OR; James W. Anderson, M.D., of the University of Kentucky; Dr. Basil M. Rifkind, chief, Lipid Metabolism and Atherogenesis Branch, National Heart, Lung and Blood Institute; Redford B. Williams, Jr., M.D., of Duke University Medical Center; David H. Blankenhorn, M.D., of the University of Southern California School of Medicine; and William H. Haskell, M.D., Ph.D., of Stanford University School of Medicine.

CONTENTS

CONTENTS

Abbreviations Used in this Book

AHA   American Heart Association

CADRF Coronary Artery Disease Risk Factor

CC   Cholesterol Cutter

CDC   Centers for Disease Control, Atlanta

mgs   milligrams

mgs/dl milligrams per deciliter

NAS   National Academy of Sciences

NCEP   National Cholesterol Education Program

NHLBI National Heart, Lung and Blood Institute

NIH   National Institutes of Health

NATURAL WAYS
TO
LOWER YOUR
CHOLESTEROL

CHAPTER ONE

How to Lower Your Cholesterol 30 Points in 30 Days

When the National Cholesterol Education Program (NCEP) announced its guidelines for desirable cholesterol levels in 1987, projections showed that more than half of all adult Americans have elevated cholesterol levels—meaning they are in the "borderline-high" or "high-risk" range. One American youngster in four also has elevated cholesterol.

The Program was launched by the National Heart, Lung and Blood Institute (NHLBI) in an effort to reduce the nation's still alarmingly high rate of death and disability from heart attack and stroke. To a great extent, these diseases are caused by excessively high deposits of cholesterol in the arteries of the heart, neck and legs. Based on cholesterol levels, the NCEP estimates that one American in four is currently at risk for heart attack or stroke during their lifetime.

Mountains of evidence exist to prove that, beyond any question of doubt or debate, the typical high-fat, high-stress, sedentary American lifestyle is the direct cause of our national high-cholesterol epidemic. It has been equally well documented that an elevated cholesterol level is directly linked to an increased risk of premature death from coronary artery disease, hypertension or stroke. Medical researchers are also finding a high cholesterol level to be an increasingly dependable indicator of potential risk for cancer, diabetes, kidney failure and similar chronic diseases which are basically caused by our affluent lifestyle.

All this has stirred Americans into a growing concern about the safety of their personal cholesterol levels. Statistics show that some 32 per cent of the population had recently taken a blood test and knew their cholesterol numbers. Nowadays, people at parties are as likely to exchange cholesterol levels as bridge scores. And most Americans continue to be hungry for information about how to lower their cholesterol and keep it low.

BEAT HIGH CHOLESTEROL WITHOUT DRUGS

Assuming your cholesterol level is elevated, this book will show you how to send your cholesterol plummetting by at least 30 points in 30 days—not by living on bean sprouts and herb teas, but by using the same safe, natural techniques taught in cholesterol clinics and cardiac rehabilitation centers. You can continue to enjoy tasty, satisfying meals without having to feel restricted or deprived.

Altogether, this book describes just about every natural, non-drug way that—directly or indirectly—is known to help lower cholesterol. There are 18 ways—more than has ever been put together in a single book or program before. Moreover, each one has been scientifically validated or medically endorsed as a dependable means of lowering cholesterol.

However, this claim is based on several conditions. First, that you are aged 21 or over. Second, that your cholesterol level is already elevated to 220 or above. Third, that you are an average American in good health, and that you realize that not all people have an identical cholesterol metabolism.

For instance, one person may experience a drop of 35 points in 30 days while another may see her cholesterol fall by only 25 points. Or one person may see her cholesterol drop 30 points in 35 days while another might achieve the same result in only 25 days. Your cholesterol may also *fail* to drop 30 points in 30 days if you continue to smoke, or are seriously overweight or diabetic.

SEND YOUR CHOLESTEROL PLUNGING DOWN

Experience has shown that the higher your cholesterol to begin with, the more rapidly it is likely to drop when you adopt, and stay with, the natural Cholesterol Cutter techniques in this book. If your cholesterol is 300, for example, it is likely to plummet a lot faster than if it is already down to 190.

Most people can lower their cholesterol to below 160. But the lower your current level, the longer it's going to take to go any lower. Typically, if you drop your cholesterol from 220 to 190 the first month and then continue to use our Cholesterol Cutter techniques, the second month might see

5

your cholesterol fall to 175, the third month to 165, and the fourth month to 160.

Although this may be the smallest, least expensive cholesterol-lowering book on the market, it is one of the few to recognize that there is more to lowering cholesterol, and to keeping it low, than a bunch of recipes for low-fat meals.

So much has been written about lowering cholesterol in the media that most of us are already aware that we can lower our cholesterol by reducing our dietary intake of cholesterol and saturated fat.

So why don't we do it?

THE NUMBERS GAME

One reason is that so many Americans have been so confused by cholesterol hype that millions have sworn never to believe another word of advice. Which is understandable when you consider that one month the American public was being told that a cholesterol level of 220 was safe while a month later, they were informed that 220 was now considered "borderline-high."

Since then, another group of top-ranking doctors has warned that no level above 160 offers total freedom from heart disease. Many people have felt so betrayed by this numbers game that they have used it as an excuse to return to their former high-risk eating habits.

Even when we *are* aware of the risks of high cholesterol, many of us are so complacent that we fail to translate our awareness into action. All too many of us have been eating and living unwisely all of our lives and we're resistant and reluctant to change. Cholesterol numbers don't mean much when we're feeling good. So we continue to eat high-risk foods and to avoid exercise.

Other millions of Americans are nutritionally illiterate. Recommendations to reduce saturated fat and cholesterol in the diet are difficult to follow if we don't know where these fats are lurking. How does 300 milligrams or 30 per cent of calories translate into actual food choices?

DRUGS OR SURGERY ARE NO PANACEA

Moreover, surveys show that many of us still believe that when the day of reckoning arrives, and an excessively high cholesterol level precipitates a heart attack or stroke, we can depend on drugs and medical treatment to bail us out.

It says a lot about our society that so many people consider it radical to replace dietary fat with fruits and vegetables, or to exercise, or to cut out smoking. Yet having a bypass or an angioplasty operation, or going on cholesterol-lowering drugs for life, is considered as normal and as American as apple pie. The same philosophy assumes that it's perfectly natural for the body to plug its arteries with cholesterol and then to self-destruct.

To a great extent, such illogical concepts arise out of mainstream medicine's focus on making mechanical repairs to the body as if it were an automobile engine. The modern mindset is to believe that, should heart disease appear, a quick cure is always available through a simple plumbing procedure called a bypass operation.

Most of us are so obsessed with hi-tech medicine that we often have unrealistic expectations of what modern medicine can actually achieve. Hi-tech or not, all that heart surgery can do is to alleviate symptoms. Unless fundamental changes in eating and living habits follow, surveys show that in the average bypass patient, half the bypass vessels may close again within 5 years. In those patients who refuse to modify their

7

health-destroying habits at all, the bypass often closes again within two or three years.

Angioplasty and atherectomy (reaming out blocked coronary arteries with, respectively, a balloon catheter, or a high-speed cutting drill) sound like cheaper alternatives. But here again, these surgical procedures may damage arteries during treatment, so much so that 30 per cent of arteries cleared by balloon angioplasty are likely to narrow again within six months.

If the thought of lowering cholesterol by natural ways turns you off, consider the alternatives. That could be either a lifetime on expensive, cholesterol-lowering drugs. Or it could very well turn into an unscheduled trip to the nearest Intensive Care Unit, possibly followed by angioplasty or a bypass operation, *plus* a lifetime on unpleasant maintenance drugs.

Nor do drugs always halt the progress of heart disease. A two-and-one-half-year survey of 120 men with severe atherosclerosis (artery-blocking cholesterol deposits) at the University of Washington, Seattle, showed that artery blockage continued to progress in 23 per cent of the men despite their taking daily cholesterol-lowering drugs.

Taking these drugs isn't most people's idea of fun, either. Some drugs taste gritty and unpleasant; they must be taken at least once daily, and they cost from $500-$2,000 annually. Adverse side effects may range from abdominal pain, gas, and bloating to constipation, headaches, fatigue, and possible liver damage. To trade lower cholesterol for these side effects is to simply replace one set of problems with another. Meanwhile, a bypass operation incurs all the risks of major surgery and even after recovery, a significant proportion of patients are never able to return to work.

It is widespread national concern about the disturbing side effects and the high cost of cholesterol-lowering drugs that has renewed interest in non-drug ways to lower cholesterol.

8

A PRUDENT DIET MAY NOT BE ENOUGH

Mainstream medicine's approach to lowering cholesterol is exemplified in the guidelines of the National Cholesterol Education Program (NCEP) and American Heart Association (AHA).

National Cholesterol Education Program Guidelines

For people aged 21 and over, the NCEP ranks cholesterol levels as:
199 and under—normal or "desirable"
200-239—borderline-high
240 and over—high risk
(Dietary changes are also suggested for those under 21 with a cholesterol level above 175).

For people with cholesterol levels of 200 or above, the AHA recommends what it calls the Prudent Diet. Step One of this lifestyle program calls for: reducing dietary fat from an average of 40 per cent of calories, as in the typical U.S. diet, to only 30 per cent or less; maintaining saturated fat intake at ten per cent or less of total calories; limiting dietary cholesterol to 100 milligrams (mgs) per 1,000 calories—or to a maximum of 300 mgs daily; stopping smoking; and exercising moderately.

For those with more seriously elevated cholesterol, or for those who fail to lower their cholesterol after six months on Step One, a slightly stricter Step Two is recommended. This calls for reducing saturated fat to six to seven per cent or less of total calories; reducing total fat to 25 per cent or less of total calories; and reducing cholesterol intake to 200 mgs or less per day.

The AHA's Step Two program compares closely to the Ideal Diet recommended several years ago by the prestigious

9

National Academy of Sciences (NAS). The NAS recommended cutting saturated fat to a maximum of 7-8 per cent of calories or less, and keeping cholesterol intake below 200-250 mgs per day.

Since nearly half of all heart attacks occur in people with cholesterol levels under 220, some researchers have criticized the NCEP's desirable cholesterol levels as being too high and their recommended dietary changes as being merely cosmetic.

To lower cholesterol further, however, requires cutting out more fat from the diet. As a result, most doctors, as well as the large health advisory agencies, believe that the American public is unwilling to accept any further reduction in dietary fats. And to point out that the NCEP's "desirable" cholesterol range of 199 or under still entails a 20 per cent risk of having a heart attack would seriously strain the public's confidence in the national cholesterol-lowering program.

THE TWO FACES OF MEDICINE

Few people realize that there are two sides to medical science. On one side is mainstream medicine, led primarily by profit-making hospitals, doctors and pharmaceutical manufacturers. At best, any type of mainstream medical treatment is likely to be impersonal, unpleasant and expensive. Far from being a permanent cure, most treatments for heart disease or stroke amount to little more than a quick fix-and-patch job.

A bypass operation cannot possibly reverse all the damage done by years of high-fat foods, stress, smoking and sedentary living. Moreover, according to a recent Rand Corporation study of common surgical procedures, researchers concluded that 30 per cent of bypass surgeries were of debatable value and 14 per cent were unjustified (cost: $37,000 to $100,000 each including surgery, hospital and drug costs, follow-up visits and rehabilitation.)

In the same study, 32 per cent of carotid endarterectomies (removing cholesterol deposits from neck arteries to prevent stroke) were also found of debatable value, and the majority were also unjustified (cost: $9,000 each). Additionally, there exists a high risk of becoming infected while in any U.S. hospital.

WHOLE PERSON HEALING
TAMES CHOLESTEROL WITHOUT DRUGS

By comparison, preventive medicine, the other side of medical science, has been far more successful. Preventive medicine is concerned with learning how to live a healthy, active life while remaining free of the same chronic diseases that mainstream medicine endeavors to treat.

In recent years, preventive medicine has made such spectacular progress that we already know how to remain healthy and to keep our cholesterol at safe and optimal levels without having to resort to drugs or surgery.

In large measure, the phenomenal success of preventive medicine is due to its Whole Person or Holistic approach. Unlike mainstream medicine, which fails to explore beyond physical symptoms, preventive medicine considers every aspect of body, mind, values, emotional stress and even spiritual beliefs. In the area of cholesterol and heart disease, at least, preventive medicine has made a mockery of many forms of mainstream medicine.

Since 1987, for instance, revolutionary new research has

11

sent shock waves through the medical community. Landmark studies, both from the field of anthropology as well as from preventive medical science, have forever changed the way many doctors view cholesterol. Breakthrough studies like the China Health Study and Dr. Dean Ornish's Lifestyle Heart Trial, have threatened to make bypass operations and cholesterol-lowering drugs almost obsolete.

The Evidence from Anthropology

In 1988, both British and American anthropologists announced that some 99 per cent of man's genes were identical to those of the chimpanzee and other higher primates. Until eight million years ago, both man and the primates shared the same common ancestor.

Until modern man appeared some 35,000 years ago, our ancestors lived primarily on coarse plant foods generally gathered by women. Men hunted, of course. But man was never quite the "great hunter" we have always assumed. Recent studies of surviving hunter-gatherer societies showed that, even with the aid of modern snares and bows and arrows, man is an inefficient procurer of meat for the table. Until comparatively recently, all meat consisted of lean wild game extremely low in artery-clogging cholesterol and saturated fat. It wasn't until the 1880s that fresh meat, eggs, cheese and sugar became widely available in stores.

Most of our genes evolved during 60 million years of life as arboreal primates. We may have lost our tails and hair and achieved flatter faces. But many anthropologists doubt that our organs have changed significantly since paleolithic times. Today, from the eyebrows down, we have inherited the physiology of a plant-eating higher primate. The DNA in each of our cells evolved out of meeting the needs of a physically-active lifestyle spent seeking fruits and other plant foods in a primeval forest.

Anthropologists point out that our digestive enzymes—our molars for grinding in place of the claws and fangs of a predator—and our long digestive tract and kidneys, all confirm that our genes were selected to equip man to thrive on plant-based foods.

Saturated fat and cholesterol hardly existed in our ancestors' diets. The result is that modern man never developed the ability to metabolize the excessive amounts of fat and cholesterol in the modern diet. However, since cholesterol is essential to human health, our livers were programmed to meet all our requirements by synthesizing some 1,500 mgs of cholesterol per day from nutrients in our traditional near-vegetarian diet.

The result is that humans have very little need for additional fat or cholesterol. Thus, when we eat the modern, fat-laden American diet, we overload our bodies with two to three times as much saturated fat and cholesterol as we can comfortably tolerate. Instead of remaining at the optimal level of 120-160, as in most plant-eating people, our cholesterol level soars to an unhealthy 215 or more. And studies show that when our cholesterol level remains that high for an extended period, deposits of surplus cholesterol appear in the arteries, choking off blood flow to heart and brain, and creating a serious risk of heart attack or stroke.

By contrast, when we eat and live as our ancestors did, our cholesterol remains at 160 or below, our arteries stay clean and clear, and coronary artery disease is unknown.

The Evidence from China

Next to rock medical science on its heels was the China Health Study, a joint effort by Cornell University, England's Oxford University, and China's Academy of Preventive Medicine. From 1983 until 1989, top researchers like Cornell's nutritional biochemist Colin Campbell, and England's Richard Peto, studied the diets and disease states of 6,500 Chinese.

They found that most rural Chinese eat the traditional plant-based diet of their ancestors while the level of physical activity is many times greater than in the West. Compared to the standard American diet, which derives 40 per cent of its calories from fat, in China only 15-20 per cent of calories come from fat. And compared to a meager 45 per cent of calories from carbohydrates, as in the American diet—most of it from low-fiber white bread and sugar—the Chinese obtain 77 per cent of their calories from carbohydrates, mostly from high-fiber fruits, vegetables, and grains. A typical day's food for a person in South China might include 19 ounces of rice, eight ounces of greens and vegetables, four ounces of starchy tubers, and less than two ounces of meat or poultry. Dairy foods are rarely seen. Combined with active exercise, a diet like this provides a lifestyle that very closely resembles that of our primate ancestors.

Hence researchers were not really surprised when the average cholesterol level in China turned out to be a healthy 127, while the rate of heart disease for males is one-sixteenth that in the U.S. The study also found that, as people in China move from a traditional diet and active lifestyle to a western diet high in saturated fat and cholesterol, and with less opportunity for physical exertion, their cholesterol levels soar and their risk for heart disease, cancer, diabetes and similar diseases of affluence increases in proportion.

Of the five billion people on this planet, four billion have cholesterol levels estimated below 160. They happen to all live in China or other Third World countries, and they follow a lifestyle and eat a diet far closer to that for which our genes evolved.

Cholesterol levels below 160—which are considered normal in most of the world—are regarded as abnormally low in the U.S., and are attainable by only five to ten per cent of the population. In most Third World countries, body levels of fat, cholesterol and blood pressure remain at the same low levels throughout life while in the U.S., they increase steadily with age. Even among the elderly, fitness is the norm in Third World countries, and youngsters are invariably lean and fit. Surprisingly while the Chinese consume an average of 20 per cent more calories per day than Americans, obesity is virtually unknown. That is because the Chinese calories come from low-fat plant foods rather than high-fat animal foods.

Conclusions from the China Health Study were that when we blend the low-fat, high-fiber diet and active lifestyle found in Third World countries with the sanitation, refrigeration, and medical care that already exist in western societies, we have the ideal conditions in which man can thrive—an environment close to that in which our ancestors evolved—and a way of life in which the average cholesterol level stays under 160, and in which everyone's arteries remain youthfully clean.

The Evidence from Preventive Medicine

In 1989, hard evidence began to appear suggesting that not only could high cholesterol be easily lowered by natural means, but that when cholesterol is kept at a level of 150 or lower for a year or more, gradual regression of existing artery-blocking cholesterol plaque takes place. The first scientifically-measured reversal of heart disease in history was confirmed in 1989 when Dean Ornish, M.D., director of the Preventive Medicine Research Institute in San Francisco, released the results of his Lifestyle Heart Trial at the American Heart Association Convention in New Orleans.

Ornish and his colleague, Larry Scherwitz, M.D., Ph.D., divided 48 heart disease patients into two groups. The control group of 20 patients followed a diet and lifestyle very similar to that recommended by the AHA. The 28 others, assigned to the optimal lifestyle group, adopted a routine that included eating an almost exclusively plant-based diet, walking briskly 3 times a week for 30 minutes, ceasing to smoke, and reducing stress through relaxation techniques—in other words, a completely comprehensive Whole Person approach.

Participants could eat as much as they liked, but only seven per cent of calories were from fat while cholesterol was limited to virtually zero. In short, their optimal lifestyle program closely resembled the lifestyle of our ancestors and of the people in rural China today.

After only a week, several of the experimental group found their angina had diminished, and a few weeks later, 90 per cent reported a noticeable decrease in heart pain. Some of those unable to walk a block at the start were soon able to walk several brisk miles. Everyone in the group felt enormously better.

As the study progressed, changes in artery diameter were periodically measured by sophisticated quantitative angiography CAT scans. After one year, measurements showed an average increase in artery diameter of 2.2 per cent. That may not sound like much but it represents an increase of 40 per cent in blood flow to the heart. Several patients were able to double blood flow to their hearts. In two patients, arteries that had been totally blocked reopened. Several of the group lost 40-50 pounds in weight. Altogether, 82 per cent of the group showed significant improvement and some were able to return to work after a long absence. Overall, the group's total cholesterol level had fallen from an average of 215 to only 151.

Meanwhile, in the control group, which generally followed AHA recommendations, 53 per cent became worse. Artery blockage increased from an average of 42.7 per cent to 46.1 per cent. Arterial lesions continued to enlarge. Some observers concluded that the AHA recommendations were too lenient. According to this study, the AHA recommendations do lower serum cholesterol. But they merely slow the progress of atherosclerosis (cholesterol blockage) rather than halting it entirely.

WHAT IS THE IDEAL CHOLESTEROL LEVEL?

Although a cholesterol level of 160 or below seems abnormally low by mainstream medical standards, it has the support of some of America's top-rated heart disease experts. In January 1988, for instance, the National Education Panel studying "Detection, Evaluation and Treatment of High Cholesterol," for the NIH agreed that customary guidelines were far too lenient and they concluded that the ideal cholesterol level is 150-160. Based on this definition, *80 per cent of U.S. adults have elevated cholesterol.* (The study was reported in *Archives of Internal Medicine*:148; 36-39, 1988.)

Another NIH authority, Dr. Basil Rifkind, chief of Lipid Metabolism at the Atherogenesis Branch of the National Heart, Lung and Blood Institute, recently suggested that there is no safe level of cholesterol within the range commonly seen in the American public, that is, above 175. Dr. Rifkind added that it might be necessary to get cholesterol down to 150 to avoid the extra risks that accompany higher levels.

The massive government-sponsored Framingham Study has also demonstrated that heart disease risk begins when cholesterol starts to rise above the 150-160 range. And Morris Rosenthal, M.D., medical director of the Santa Monica Pritikin Center, reports that heart disease is extremely rare in anyone with a cholesterol level under 160. Even the ultra-conservative AHA advises that the cholesterol level should never exceed 200.

Out of these and similar studies has come a radical new formula for calculating the ideal cholesterol level. That formula is:

100 + your age = ideal cholesterol level

Regardless of age, however, the absolute maximum level should never exceed 160.

According to this formula, the ideal cholesterol level for any person aged 40 is 100 + 40 = 140. But for anyone aged 60 or over, the ideal maximum level remains at 160.

This formula has already been widely adopted by the majority of practitioners of preventive medicine. Even some mainstream medical practitioners have been so impressed that their cholesterol-lowering recommendations now go beyond the guidelines of the AHA and similar large health-advisory agencies.

One thing is certain, however. A level of 160 or below is seldom attainable on the liberal nutritional guidelines endorsed by the AHA and other mainstream agencies. To lower your cholesterol to really safe levels, it's necessary to adopt nutritional guidelines closer to those of Ornish's Lifestyle Heart Trial and the China Health Study.

Meanwhile, the AHA, the NAS and similar health advisory agencies point out that their recommendations generally specify *maximum* amounts. For example, they invariably recommend "a *maximum* limit of 30 per cent *or less* of calories from fat." They are also in general agreement that people who consume a total fat level *below* 30 per cent of calories (or *below* 300 mgs of cholesterol, or *below* ten per cent of calories from saturated fat) have a lower prevalence of heart disease.

OUTDISTANCING CHOLESTEROL THE NATURAL WAY

Much of the confusion and controversy surrounding the cholesterol issue is due to the existance of two very different schools of thought. The preventive medicine school is clearly showing that three times a day, the average American consumes more saturated fat and cholesterol than most people's bodies can handle. And the excess is destined to line our arteries.

Once we stop piling the fat onto our plates, allowing our cholesterol levels to drop to the 150-160 range, our arteries may actually begin to heal. Gradually, existing cholesterol deposits that are blocking the arteries begin to dissolve, and vital blood flow to the heart, brain and limbs is apparently restored.

To reach this "healing" zone usually means reducing total fat intake to 20 per cent of calories or below. By combining this dietary step with a daily walk and stress reduction techniques, tens of thousands of Americans have already seen their artery blockage gradually dissolve and their heart disease disappear.

Literally tens of thousands of cases of regression or reversal of artery-clogging atherosclerosis have been documented at the numerous cardiac rehabilitation centers which now exist across the country. When saturated fat and cholesterol are eliminated from the diet, it is considered routine for elevated cholesterol levels to plummet while angina pain often begins to diminish or disappear after only a week or two.

WHEN YOU MAY NEED
YOUR DOCTOR'S APPROVAL

At this point, we must emphasize that it is not the intent of this book to recommend that you attempt to reverse existing coronary heart disease, or any other form of disease or dysfunction, by using any of the techniques described in this book without your doctor's approval.

An essential step in the cholesterol-lowering program in this book is to take a cholesterol test *accompanied by a medical evaluation.* If you already have angina, coronary artery disease, diabetes, hypertension or any other disease, dysfunction or medical condition, you must obtain your doctor's specific permission before using any of the techniques in this book.

If you wish to lower your cholesterol into the healing zone in an attempt to reverse angina, coronary artery disease, or claudication (or any other medical condition) through the preventive medicine approach, *you should do so only under supervision of a medical doctor, preferably one who practices preventive medicine.*

THE GUARANTEED WAY TO A HEALTHIER HEART AND ARTERIES

It must be abundantly clear by now that the way to lower cholesterol is to live as closely as possible to the diet and lifestyle of our ancestors, or to the people of contemporary Third World countries such as China. Supporting this premise is the discovery that lowering cholesterol is dose-related. That is, the more Cholesterol Cutter techniques you employ, and the more faithfully you follow them, the faster your cholesterol is likely to plummet and the lower it is eventually likely to drop.

Numerous studies have shown that cholesterol will fall faster, and reach lower levels, when fat intake is reduced to 15 per cent of calories than when it is reduced to only 30 per cent. As other Cholesterol Cutter methods, such as exercise and stress-management techniques are added, the cholesterol level should drop even faster, and is capable of reaching still lower levels.

It is for this reason that the most successful cholesterol clinics and cardiac rehabilitation centers have adopted a Whole Person approach.

Although elevated cholesterol levels can be significantly lowered through dietary modification alone, the average person often has difficulty staying on a low-fat diet. Social pressure from family and friends eager to have you share their fat-loaded meals often makes compliance difficult. And millions of Americans sabotage their good intentions by using

21

fatty foods as a tranquilizer to help defuse emotional stress. Whenever they feel tense, they head for the refrigerator.

A Cholesterol Level Risk Chart
The risk chart below shows the advantages of lowering your cholesterol to various levels.

Total Cholesterol Level	
300	Risk of heart disease is 5 times as great as at the 200 level.
240	Lowest limit of NCEP's "high-risk" zone. Risk of heart disease is twice that at the 200 level.
225	Average level of U.S. heart attack victim.
213	Average level for U.S. women.
211	Average level for U.S. men.
200	Lowest limit of NCEP's "borderline-high" zone. At 200 you have half the normal U.S. risk for heart disease.
199	Upper limit of NCEP's normal or "desirable" zone.
185	Average male cholesterol level in Japan.
180	At this level and above, heart disease risk begins to appear.
170	Maximum desirable level for children based on U.S. standards.
160	Upper limit of preventive medicine's zone of total safety from coronary heart disease.
150	Upper limit of preventive medicine's "healing" zone. Below this level, risk of coronary artery disease becomes almost nonexistent.
145	Average level in most Third World countries.
127	Average level in rural China and in strict vegetarians everywhere, including the U.S.

LOWERING CHOLESTEROL REQUIRES
A WHOLE PERSON APPROACH

For these and other reasons, most practitioners of preventive medicine have concluded that high-cholesterol is a Whole Person problem, and the majority of these doctors employ an array of therapeutic options which work on every level of mind-body function.

The 18 Cholesterol Cutter techniques in this book include just about every option currently offered by the most advanced cholesterol clinics and cardiac centers across the nation. Some of our therapies function on the dietary, nutritional and physical levels while others work on the emotional and pyschological levels. This varied array of methodologies allows you to use a completely holistic approach.

In other words, you can practice preventive medicine on your own. As you read on, you will learn how you can intervene in and manipulate your own cholesterol levels, and how you can modify the components of your cholesterol, and fine-tune them, using only the natural methods in these pages.

Studies in behaviorial medicine have confirmed that most cholesterol problems are directly linked to emotional stress that is then translated into physiological mechanisms. For example, in response to emotional stress, or to the added stress of social pressures, millions of Americans have become physically addicted to fatty foods and sugar.

Thus the key to lowering cholesterol may not be simply cutting fat from the diet, but mobilizing the motivation and determination to actually do it. Virtually all of our 18 Cholesterol Cutter techniques require you to take an active role in your own recovery. In the process, they promote taking control of your life and taking responsibility for your own wellness.

23

IT'S UP TO YOU TO ACT

Merely reading this book can't change your way of eating or exercise habits or manage stress for you. Nor can it reprogram inappropriate beliefs that may be torpedoing your motivation.

Preventive medicine puts you in full control. It is up to you to play an active role. Through some of our techniques, for example, you can enter deep relaxation and use biofeedback to relax your arteries and to release much of the stress and pressure in your life.

By comparison, drugs and surgery are passive therapies. Something is done to you by a substance, or by another person, without any effort or cooperation on your part. While passive therapies have obvious uses, preventive medicine believes that they often engender feelings of hopelessness and helplessness. Thus they are used only as a last, desperate resort.

Preventive medicine, also known as holistic medicine or holistic healing, is a multidisciplinary approach that employs multimodal therapies. One of its branches is behavioral medicine. To be completely effective, preventive medicine should be practiced by a medical doctor.

Although able to prescribe powerful drugs if needed, doctors in this field prefer to minimize use of pharmaceuticals and most employ drugs only when absolutely necessary. Much preferred are harmless, drug-free therapies such as nutrition and diet, exercise, relaxation, biofeedback and stress management. Each of these active therapies are included among the Cholesterol Cutter techniques in this book.

STRAIGHTENING OUT THE CHOLESTEROL CONTROVERSY

To help separate myths and fallacies about cholesterol from scientifically validated facts and figures, the first task of this book is to help you become a medically informed layperson—at least, where cholesterol is concerned. By absorbing the information in this book, you may become almost as knowledgeable about cholesterol as your doctor is.

Naturally, such facts are presented for information only and are not intended as a substitute for your doctor's extensive training and experience. Should you require medical treatment, being a medically informed layperson will undoubtedly help you and your doctor to cooperate more closely and to work together as partners.

To become medically informed—to cut through all the conflicting information and biased advice—you must read this book all the way through. Reading about each of the 18 Cholesterol Cutters adds more to your knowledge of cholesterol and how to manage it. Thus the first step is to acquire this know-how. This is not a large book and many people are able to read it through in a single evening.

Each chapter and each technique expands your knowledge about cholesterol and adds to the numbers of therapies you can use. You can then put your knowledge to work to lower your cholesterol to safe levels.

CHAPTER TWO

How to Get an Accurate Cholesterol Test— and Interpret the Results

B efore you do a thing about lowering your cholesterol, you *must* take a cholesterol test. Only after you have taken a battery of tests for a full "Cardiovascular Risk Profile" (also called a Lipoprotein Analysis or Coronary Risk Profile) should you begin any of the Cholesterol Cutter techniques in this book.

While a simple cholesterol test at a mall or health fair may give you a rough idea of your cholesterol level, it simply doesn't reveal the information you need to fine-tune your own cholesterol.

The reason is that the overall cholesterol level—the one we've been talking about so far—actually represents the sum of three different cholesterol components. In medical terminology, the overall cholesterol level is known as the serum, plasma or blood cholesterol. It is also frequently called the Total Cholesterol because it is the sum total of the three cholesterol components in the blood stream.

These three components are known as Lipoproteins. They are necessary because cholesterol (a *lipid* or fat) can travel through the blood stream only when encased in a *protein* bubble, hence the name *lipoprotein*. (The full role played by each lipoprotein is discussed in Chapter 4.) Meanwhile, knowing the exact level of each lipoprotein fraction reveals a much clearer picture of your actual heart disease risk.

All cholesterol numbers represent milligrams per deciliter. A total cholesterol of 160 indicates 160 thousandths (or .16) of a gram of cholesterol per tenth of a liter of blood plasma. From here on, the abbreviation "mgs/dl" will accompany all cholesterol, lipoprotein and triglycerides numbers; and overall cholesterol will be referred to as "total cholesterol."

Here's how a total cholesterol of 220 mgs/dl looks when broken down into typical levels of its lipoprotein components.

Typical Percentage of Total Cholesterol	Lipoprotein Fraction	Mgs/dl
65%	LDL—Low Density Lipoprotein (bad cholesterol)	143
20%	HDL—High Density Lipoprotein (good cholesterol)	44
15%	VLDL—Very Low Density Lipoprotein (another bad cholesterol)	33
100%	Total Cholesterol	220

27

Another important indicator invariably included in a Coronary Risk Factor blood test is triglycerides (circulating blood fats). Triglycerides are also measured in mgs/dl. The triglycerides level is equal to approximately five times the VLDL level. So in this case, triglycerides would be roughly 33 × 5, or 165 mgs/dl.

HOW TO HANDLE YOUR CHOLESTEROL TEST

A cholesterol test is the next best thing to taking a look inside your arteries. By revealing the amount of cholesterol in the bloodstream, the test also indicates the degree of arterial blockage caused by cholesterol plaque (deposits).

Approximately ten cubic centimeters of blood is painlessly withdrawn from a vein in your arm. At the lab, your blood is spun in a centrifuge to separate out the cells. Then a sample of serum is analyzed by a special machine. It may be one or two days before you are given the results.

Although you may save a few dollars by having a lab analyze your blood and give you a printout, we strongly recommend that for your initial test, you work through your family doctor or through an internist or general practitioner. Ideally, choose a physician who is sympathetic to preventive medicine. Avoid any physician who is overweight or flabby, or who smokes and doesn't exercise, or who overmedicalizes everything and tends to prescribe a drug solution for every problem.

You need a competent physician to evaluate your initial cholesterol test in order to screen out any possibility of a medical problem such as heart disease, hypertension, diabetes, or familial hypercholesterolemia, which could be life-threatening if not diagnosed. You may also need medical clearance before commencing any diet change or exercise program. Tell your doctor about all the natural techniques in this book that you contemplate using and have him give you medical clearance to practice them.

Depending on your condition, the doctor may also want to include other tests, such as an exercise electrocardiogram (EKG) test or a glucose value. If you have any disease or dysfunction of the intestines or bowels, or a bowel disorder or kidney disease, or if you could possibly develop a blocked bowel, or have had recent surgery, get your doctor's approval before increasing fiber intake.

In most cases, it is appreciably cheaper to handle everything through one physician in a single visit. Frequently, it can all be done for $75 to $125, including a full Cardiovascular Risk Profile cholesterol test. Many people find their insurance pays for the whole thing.

Once you have your doctor's OK, you can have any subsequent tests made directly through a lab. However, once you have consulted a physician for an initial cholesterol test, he or she will usually arrange subsequent tests without any additional consulting fee.

Make sure, before going ahead with any specific doctor, that he or she very clearly agrees to give you a photocopy of your complete lab report, with every figure and result included. You need these figures to make your own risk assessment (in addition to any assessment made by your doctor). Never settle for a verbal test result.

HAVE YOUR TEST ANALYZED
BY A CALIBRATED LAB

Try to avoid having your specimen analyzed in a doctor's lab. Instead, have it sent to a calibrated lab, preferably one calibrated by the National Institutes of Health. If the lab is also certified by the American College of Pathologists, or the Centers for Disease Control, so much the better. Ask about the lab's built-in error rate. It should not exceed five per cent. Most hospital labs are calibrated and results are more dependable.

Careful lab selection is necessary because several recent university studies have found that in many run-of-the-mill labs, faulty specimen preparation, inaccurate instrument preparation, and unskilled operators are all too common. Furthermore, your own cholesterol level isn't always stable. Biological variation due to stress, weight change, the menstrual cycle, illness, or medications can cause your personal cholesterol level to fluctuate by as much as 10-13 per cent.

Due to a combination of these factors, it's not unusual for a cholesterol reading to be off by as much as 15 per cent. This means that a person with a "desirable" total cholesterol of 190 mgs/dl could be falsely diagnosed as having a level of 218, placing her in the "borderline-high" range. Or a person with a level of 211 mgs/dl (borderline-high) could be classed as 241 (high-risk). Conversely, a person in the high-risk zone might be classified as only borderline-high.

MINIMIZING ERRORS
IN YOUR CHOLESTEROL TEST

The following precautions can help minimize any possibility of error. Avoid taking a cholesterol test when you have a viral infection. Women should avoid the test during the last days of the menstrual cycle, or if pregnant. Cholesterol levels rise during pregnancy so it's best to wait three or four months after giving birth. Medications such as beta-blockers, diuretics, and birth control pills, or estrogen or progesterone, may also affect test results. If you are taking any of these, or any medication for that matter, consult your physician before taking a cholesterol test.

For any test which measures lipoprotein fractions or triglycerides, you must fast for 12-14 hours beforehand—usually from 6 p.m. the previous evening. You'll also get a more accurate result if you refrain from any vigorous activity during the same period. Lipoprotein fractions are calculated by a formula based on triglycerides. And triglycerides are affected by recent food intake. Hence the necessity to fast and stay relaxed.

When taking the actual test, insist on sitting down for 10-15 minutes beforehand to allow body fluids to pool, and remain seated during the test. Insist also that blood is drawn from a vein in the arm, and is *not* taken from a prick in the finger. Fingerprick samples draw blood from the capilleries and are notoriously inaccurate. Your tester should don a fresh pair of gloves for each person, and your arm should be disinfected first. Once taken, the specimen should be analyzed fairly promptly. It should not have to be stored for any length of time prior to analysis.

Although it takes five or six weeks for cholesterol levels to stabilize after a diet or lifestyle change, you can get a fairly good indication by taking a second test after 30 days on our Cholesterol Cutter techniques.

DAVID McBRAYNE DROPS HIS CHOLESTEROL 31 POINTS IN 30 DAYS

David McBrayne, a hard-working 45-year-old Chicago stockbroker, loved rich meats and creamy desserts and his waistline showed it. After weeks of pleading, his wife persuaded him to visit his doctor for a cholesterol test. When the results came back, they looked like this.

David's "Before" Test

Percentage of Total Cholesterol	Lipoprotein Fractions	Mgs/dl
65	LDL—"bad" cholesterol	156
20	HDL—"good" cholesterol	48
15	VLDL—another "bad" cholesterol	36
100	Total Cholesterol	240

Triglycerides: approximately 180

The doctor's eyebrows shot up when he saw the test results. David was immediately placed on a combined eating and exercise plan very similar to that of the Chol-Tamer Plan described later in this book.

Thirty days later, after a second cholesterol test, the results came back looking like this:

32

David's "After" Test

Percentage of Total Cholesterol	Lipoprotein Fractions	Mgs/dl
62	LDL—"bad" cholesterol	129
24	HDL—"good" cholesterol	50
14	VLDL—another "bad" cholesterol	30
100	Total Cholesterol	209

Triglycerides: approximately 150

Not only had David's total cholesterol dropped by 31 mgs/dl but his two "bad" cholesterols had also fallen significantly. Meanwhile, his "good" cholesterol had increased slightly. Furthermore, the proportion of LDL, the "bad" cholesterol, had dropped from 65 to 62 per cent while that of VLDL, another "bad" cholesterol, had slipped from 15 to 14 percent.

Triglycerides, or blood fats, had also fallen from 180 mgs/dl to only 150. Simultaneously, the proportion of good cholesterol rose from 20 to 24 per cent.

We must briefly explain here that we need more of the "good" cholesterol because HDL carries surplus cholesterol out of the arteries and back to the liver where it is excreted. We need less, much less, LDL, the "bad" cholesterol, because LDL brings cholesterol from the liver and tends to dump it into the arteries where it can form plaque and block blood flow to the heart, brain and limbs. By the same token, we also need fewer VLDLs and a lower level of triglycerides.

Don't worry if your HDL drifts down a few points rather than rising slightly as David's did. When both total cholesterol and LDL undergo steep drops, it's typical for the HDL to lose a few points also. However, LDL typically drops 3-4 times as much as HDL.

33

FINE TUNING CHOLESTEROL LEVELS

As David did, it is relatively easy to manipulate your lipo-protein fractions by intervening with the Cholesterol Cutter techniques in this book.

Reducing the amount of saturated fat, total fat and choles-terol in the diet should cause an immediate drop in LDL levels, and also in triglycerides. When triglycerides fall, fewer VLDLs are needed to carry them through the bloodstream, and VLDL levels also drop.

HDL levels are suppressed by a sedentary lifestyle, cigarette smoking, a high degree of stress, being overweight and hav-ing a high proportion of body fat. A combination of stress and smoking can take the HDL as low as 25-30 mgs/dl—a dangerously low level for most Americans.

HDL rises when all of these counter-productive habits are eliminated and we do the very opposite. HDL rises in re-sponse to regular aerobic exercise, and to losing weight and body fat, managing stress and ceasing to smoke. Many of our 18 Cholesterol Cutter techniques are designed to achieve exactly this.

Admittedly, it is easier to lower total cholesterol and LDL by reducing dietary fat than it is to raise HDL by exercise. Nonetheless, when a low-fat diet is combined with an aero-bic exercise program, and with other health-restoring tech-niques in this book, levels of total and LDL cholesterol both plunge while HDL tends to rise.

To reach and stay below a total cholesterol level of 160 mgs/dl usually requires reducing total fat intake to ten per cent of dietary calories, or slightly less. By manipulating diet, exercise and other lifestyle factors, we ourselves can attain almost any desired combination of total cholesterol, LDL,

HDL, VLDL and triglycerides. In the process, we can reach a level of wellness so high that heart disease is virtually non-existant.

HOW TO READ YOUR
CHOLESTEROL TEST PRINTOUT

When it arrives from the lab, your cholesterol test printout could look something like this.

	Result	Normal Values in Mgs/dl
Total Cholesterol	230	desirable: 199 or under borderline-high 200-239 elevated: 240 or over
LDL Cholesterol	150	desirable: 129 or below borderline: 130-159 elevated: 160 or over
HDL Cholesterol	46	male 30-75 female 40-90
Triglycerides	170	30-150

The VLDL level is often not shown. That's because you can easily calculate it yourself by subtracting the sum of LDL and HDL from the total cholesterol. (Example: 230 − [150 + 46] = 34.)

What, exactly, do the levels of your lipoproteins and triglycerides indicate?

LDL—The "Bad" Cholesterol

LDL is a major indicator of heart disease risk and the lower the level the better. For optimal health, LDL should be under 100 mgs/dl. A range of 100-130 mgs/dl is considered acceptable if you have only one other risk for heart disease. Levels between 130-160 mgs/dl are borderline and become high-risk in association with two other risk factors for heart disease. Any level from 160 mgs/dl on up is considered a serious health risk.

When LDL tops 160 mgs/dl (or 130 in association with two other risk factors) most physicians recommend six months of treatment with diet and exercise. If this fails, drugs may be prescribed.

HDL—The "Good" Cholesterol

The higher your HDL the better. For every ten mgs increase in HDL, heart disease risk is estimated to fall by 50 per cent. In males, HDL can range from 30-75 mgs/dl and, in Americans, averages 45. In females, HDL can range from 40-90 mgs/dl and, in Americans, averages 55. Anyone who eats the standard American diet is generally safe when HDL is over 45 mgs/dl while a high of 70-80 is considered optimal.

How risky is it to have an HDL level of, say, 35 mgs/dl or below? The answer seems to depend on the levels of your total cholesterol and LDL. In America, where doctors see few people with a total cholesterol of 160 mgs/dl or under, an HDL below 35 is generally regarded as a risk factor for developing heart disease. Confirming this widely-held view is a report issued in February 1992 by a National Institutes of Health panel, stating that if the total cholesterol is 200 mgs/dl or above, an HDL below 35 constitutes a high risk factor for developing coronary artery disease.

However, over 60 per cent of the world's population eats a primarily plant-based diet and in these people a total cholesterol of 160 mgs/dl or below is regarded as commonplace. Frequently, such people also have an LDL of under 100 mgs/dl accompanied by an HDL of under 35.

The explanation is that at these low levels, there really isn't much surplus cholesterol for HDLs to carry out of the arteries, hence the need for a high HDL level is much less than in meat-eating Americans. Thus, within these parameters, an HDL below 35 mgs/dl seems to imply little or no added risk. In vegetarians, and in many third world peoples, HDL often ranges between 25 and 35 mgs/dl while these people are virtually immune from most of the chronic diseases that wipe out older Americans.

As a result, some practitioners of preventive medicine in the U.S. now consider that, in persons with a total cholesterol of 160 mgs/dl or below, the HDL level is safe provided it is at least 21 per cent of the total cholesterol level. (Example: a total cholesterol level of 150 mgs/dl with an HDL of 32 is considered safe because the HDL exceeds 21 per cent of total cholesterol.)

VLDL—Another "Bad" Cholesterol

Although VLDL particles carry about ten per cent of all cholesterol, each also carries five times its own weight of triglycerides. After dumping its triglyceride load in body cells, and becoming fat-depleted, VLDLs are transformed into LDLs. Generally, the lower your VLDL level, the better.

VLDL levels are considered acceptable up to 30 mgs/dl;

or up to 20 if you have a genetic history of heart disease, if you have one or more risk factors for heart disease, or if you are a woman over 60 with a total cholesterol of 200 or more.

Triglycerides

Regrettably, many doctors still overlook triglycerides when ordering a lipoprotein analysis while few physicians concur on what constitutes a high level. However, recent research—of which your doctor may be unaware—leaves no doubt about triglycerides levels and where risk begins.

The normal range of triglycerides is considered to be 30-135 mgs/dl.

100 or under is excellent
120 or below is desirable in men (in women, levels should be lower still)
120-149 is considered borderline
150 or above is considered high by Framingham Heart Study researchers
150-249 can constitute a risk to health
250-499 is considered dangerously high
500-1000 or above can lead to life-threatening pancreatitis.
Any reading over 1000 calls for immediate drug therapy.

In men, most doctors still do not consider a high triglycerides level by itself as a risk factor for heart disease. But in women, triglycerides are often a better predictor of heart disease risk than in men. In either sex, a level of 150 mgs/dl or higher is nowadays considered a signal to see your physician. Almost always it is due to some kind of lipid abnormality that could heighten risk of heart disease.

All too often, the abnormality consists of an excessive dietary intake of fat from animal or tropical oil sources. Such an overload impairs the liver's ability to break down fat, allowing the surplus to enter the bloodstream as triglycerides. To make things worse, the high fat intake also triggers the liver to overproduce cholesterol.

A borderline-to-high triglyceride level is also often due to being 20 per cent or more overweight and/or consuming 1-2 ounces or more of alcohol daily. Levels of 250 mgs/dl or above may also be due to diabetes, medications or diseases of the liver, kidneys or thyroid gland.

To avoid the obvious risks of high triglycerides, you should always ask your doctor to specifically include triglycerides in your lipoprotein analysis.

It was Framingham Heart Study researchers who first defined triglycerides as high if over 150 mgs/dl and that a desirable level should be under 120 and lower still in women. Levels below 100 are considered excellent but in the U.S. are usually found only in devout Mormons and Seventh Day Adventists, and in vegetarians and others who eat a diet in which not more than ten per cent of calories are from fat.

A good general rule is that the more fat you eat, the higher your triglycerides. Refined carbohydrates (white flour, sugar and alcohol) can also indirectly raise your triglycerides. To lower triglycerides, weight loss is very effective as is physical exercise and a diet high in fiber and low in fat (fewer than 10-20 per cent of calories from fat).

Caution: if your triglycerides are over 150 mgs/dl and your HDL is under 40, you may be at serious risk for heart disease. This can be true even if your total cholesterol is under 200 mgs/dl. In this case, you should lose no time in consulting a physician.

A BETTER ASSESSMENT OF YOUR CHOLESTEROL RISK

To help put the lipoprotein levels into perspective in assessing your actual risk of coronary artery disease, most cardiologists evaluate the 4 Coronary Artery Disease Risk Factors (CADRF)

CADRF #1

Factor #1 is the total cholesterol level alone. The range of levels for total cholesterol were discussed in full in Chapter 1. Mainstream medicine considers a level of 199 mgs/dl or below to be "desirable," 200-239 to be "borderline-high" and 240 up to be "high-risk" or elevated. The preventive medicine school considers that any level above 160 mgs/dl implies some risk while at levels below 150, assuming no other risk factors are present, coronary artery disease ceases to be a hazard to human health.

CADRF #2

Factor #2 is the LDL level alone. Since LDL is relatively easy to lower by diet, it is considered an important predictor of heart disease risk in adults. When the total cholesterol level drops, most of the reduction takes place in the LDL fraction. LDL levels are rated thus:

100 mgs/dl or under: ideal.
100-130 mgs/dl: acceptable
130-160 mgs/dl: borderline.
161 mgs/dl or above: at risk.

40

CADRF #3

When total cholesterol levels are between 160 and 250 mgs/dl, the ratio between total cholesterol and HDL is considered an important indicator of heart disease, especially in older people. Several studies have found that when total cholesterol level are between 200 and 240 mgs/dl, this ratio can predict your heart disease risk three to four times more accurately than the LDL level alone, and five to six times more accurately than the total cholesterol level alone.

Framingham Heart Study researchers also found this ratio extremely helpful in evaluating heart disease risk in people with a total cholesterol level above 160 mgs/dl. However, the ratio becomes insignificant when total cholesterol is 150 mgs/dl or lower and it also does not work as well when total cholesterol is 250 or above.

By way of illustration let's examine this ratio in the case of David's *Before* and *After* tests.

$$\text{Before: } \frac{\text{total cholesterol}}{\text{HDL}} \text{ or } \frac{240}{48} = 5$$

$$\text{After: } \frac{\text{total cholesterol}}{\text{HDL}} \text{ or } \frac{210}{50} = 4.2$$

Ratios are classed as:

3.5 and below is ideal
3.5–4 is good
4.1–4.6 is fair
4.7–5.25 is poor
5.3 and above may indicate heart disease risk

Thus David's *Before* ratio of 5 indicated that he was at some risk. But after 30 days of using cholesterol-lowering techniques, his ratio had fallen to a much safer 4.2.

A level of 3.5 or below generally indicates you are safe from coronary artery disease. However, Framingham Heart Study researchers found that even at ratios between 3.5 and 4.5, atherosclerosis plaque will still slowly accumulate in the arteries. If you live long enough, it may eventually cause lesions in the coronary arteries.

Incidentally, the national average ratio for men is a not-so-good 5 and for women 4.4 Because women's HDL is usually higher than men's, women generally have a lower ratio.

This ratio will immediately reveal a serious heart disease risk. Consider, for example, a person with a total cholesterol of 220 mgs/dl and an HDL of only 32. The ratio is:

$$\frac{\text{total cholesterol}}{\text{HDL}} \text{ or } \frac{220}{32} = 6.8$$

CADRF #4

This factor is the ratio between LDL and HDL (LDL divided by HDL). In David's case, the *Before* and *After* ratios were:

$$\text{Before: } \frac{\text{LDL}}{\text{HDL}} \text{ or } \frac{156}{48} = 3.25$$

$$\text{After: } \frac{\text{LDL}}{\text{HDL}} \text{ or } \frac{130}{50} = 2.6$$

Desirable ratios should be 3 or less. Hence David made significant progress in lowering his ratio from 3.25 to only 2.6.

Generally, vegetarians and exercise enthusiasts show the best LDL/HDL ratios while smokers have the worst. Women typically have lower ratios than men.

Assessing David's Ultimate Cholesterol Risk

Taken together, David's 4 CADRF factors looked like this:

	Before	After	Difference
#1, total cholesterol	240	210	-30
#2, LDL	156	130	-26
#3, chol/HDL ratio	5	4.2	-.8
#4, LDL/HDL ratio	3.25	2.6	-.65
Triglycerides	180	150	-30

This overall assessment indicates that David's total cholesterol fell from being "high-risk" to being only "borderline-high"; his LDL dropped from borderline to acceptable; his total cholesterol/HDL ratio rose from poor to fair; his LDL/HDL ratio fell from an undesirable 3.25 to a desirable 2.6; and his triglycerides dropped from high to normal.

These simple formulas can help you make an accurate assessment of your coronary artery disease risk. They will also reveal exactly how much real progress you have made between your first cholesterol test and the second.

Naturally, there is no pressing need to take a second test to see how you're doing *exactly* 30 days after you begin this program. Unless your doctor recommends a second test at a specific time, you could, if you wished, easily wait 60 or even 90 days before taking your second cholesterol test.

CHOLESTEROL ISN'T THE WHOLE STORY

It may come as something of a shock at this point to realize that, after having learned to make a full and complete assessment of your coronary artery disease risk due to cholesterol deposits, cholesterol is merely one of a number of risk factors for heart disease.

In addition to elevated cholesterol, at least 12 other risk factors exist for heart disease. Having several of these other risk factors, such as hypertension, obesity, and smoking *could* lead to a heart attack even if your total cholesterol is under 180 mgs/dl.

A low cholesterol level safeguards you only from coronary artery disease, a condition almost invariably due to blockage of arteries by cholesterol deposits. However, a heart attack, stroke, painful angina, or intermittent claudication in the legs, can also be caused by smoking or by having a hostile and cynical personality.

While high cholesterol levels are primarily caused by a high-fat diet and an unhealthy sedentary lifestyle, these counter-productive habits may also be the cause of other heart disease risk factors such as obesity, hypertension, and Type II diabetes.

Fortunately, most body functions are so inter-related that when you adopt a Whole Person approach to lowering cholesterol, certain other heart disease risk factors may disappear along with the elevated cholesterol. The 18 Cholesterol Cutter techniques in this book should have a powerfully beneficial effect on Whole Person health.

So let's take a look at each of these 12 other multiple risk factors.

Gender

Hormone production protects most women from heart disease before menopause (except when diabetes or smoking is present). But after age 60, women have the same heart disease risk as men. After age 60, cholesterol levels are a more accurate predictor of heart disease risk in women than they are in men.

Age

With rising age, men show a linear increase in heart disease risk. All other things being equal, a man of 70 has twice the heart disease risk of a man of 50.

Until recently, it was also thought that at age 65 and over, cholesterol levels had diminishing influence on heart disease risk. But recent findings from the Honolulu Heart Program changed all that. After following 1,480 men aged 65 and over for 12 years, the authors concluded that elevated cholesterol levels were a dependable predictor of heart disease risk for *all* older people, both men and women. Regardless of age, they found that risk of heart disease rises two per cent for every one per cent rise in total cholesterol. In fact, the older you become, the greater the impact of cholesterol. So don't let advancing years deter you from getting a cholesterol test.

One American child in four also has an elevated cholesterol level. This is because most American children are permitted to eat just about anything they desire with little or no

45

nutritional guidance. While elevated cholesterol in children can be inherited, it is also common in families with no genetic predisposition.

Actual risk of adult heart disease from elevated cholesterol levels in children remains controversial. The Bogalusa Heart Study found that children with the highest cholesterol levels tended to have the highest levels as adults. But other studies have indicated that in 56 per cent of boys and over 70 per cent of girls with elevated cholesterol, the levels normalize in adulthood.

Thus the American Academy of Pediatricians recommends cholesterol tests only for children with a family history of premature heart disease. However, most authorities agree that children over six with elevated cholesterol should be placed on a low-fat diet. Agreement is also virtually unanimous that all children should be tested on reaching puberty to screen out anyone with a genetic tendency to high cholesterol.

Diabetes

Type II, or adult-onset, diabetes is a strong risk factor for heart disease. It offsets the protection provided to women by female hormones, and creates heart disease risk prior to menopause. A high blood insulin level also stimulates the liver to produce more cholesterol.

High Blood Pressure

Hypertension, or high blood pressure, can damage arteries and cause plaque to build up. Have your blood pressure taken along with your cholesterol test. If your level exceeds 140/90, ask your physician for advice.

Enlargement of Left Ventricle

This condition is a frequent forerunner of angina pain and heart disease. If your doctor suspects this condition, he can check you out with an EKG test at the same time that your cholesterol test is being evaluated.

If you have any history of transient ischemic attacks, stroke, intermittent claudication or angina, you should discuss these risk factors with your doctor during the visit.

Genetic Predisposition to High Cholesterol

Due to one of several genetic factors, entire families may have premature coronary artery disease. If one of your biological relatives has had premature heart disease (before age 55), you could also be at early risk for heart disease.

The most common inherited high-cholesterol condition is familial hypercholesterolemia. Most people with a total cholesterol of 400 or higher have this dysfunction. A person with a total cholesterol of 500 mgs/dl., and no other risk factors, has a 30 per cent chance of a heart attack within the next seven years.

Familial hypercholesterolemia results from having an extremely low count of LDL and HDL receptors in body cells. When cholesterol-carrying LDL particles are unable to bind to LDL receptors in body cells, they dump their cholesterol load in the arteries where it can build up into an atherosclerotic deposit and block blood flow.

An Inactive or Sedentary Lifestyle

Most heart disease risk appraisals overlook the benefits of exercise in reducing heart disease risk. Steven N. Blair, P.E.D., director of epidemiology at the Institute of Aerobics Research in Dallas, believes all multi-risk appraisals should regard an inactive or sedentary lifestyle as a major risk factor for heart disease and other chronic diseases. A long-term study at the Institute recently showed that a person with a low level of fitness had twice the risk of dying from a degenerative disease as a person who is moderately fit.

Tendency of Blood to Clot

One result of eating a diet high in fat is that blood platelets coagulate more readily. This raises the risk of heart attack or stroke due to a blood clot. Mainstream medicine's answer is to take an aspirin every other day. But aspirin simply alleviates symptoms without addressing the underlying cause. Risk of a blood clot can be significantly reduced by following the advice in Cholesterol Cutters (CCs) #2 through 13.

Hostile Type-A Behavior

Frequently found in time-pressured Type-A personalities, free-floating hostility, together with anger, rage or cynicism, can create a major stress risk factor for high cholesterol and heart disease. These self-destructive emotions can be defused by following the recommendations in CCs #16, 17 and 18.

Obesity

Obesity implies being 30 per cent or more overweight and constitutes a major risk factor for heart disease. Recent studies have also shown that when surplus weight exists as a paunch, or as a belly spilling out over the belt, this may be a possible diagnostic indicator of a high level of cholesterol and lipids, and of added risk for all chronic disease.

Overweight men tend to have bellies or paunches and to be apple-shaped, while women tend to carry their surplus weight on the hips and thighs, which makes them pear-shaped. Being apple-shaped is considered a greater health risk than being pear-shaped. Many apple-shaped men also tend to be stocky, to exhibit male-pattern baldness and also to have tell-tale patches of fat under the eyes, or on the Achilles tendons, and on the backs of the hands. Some researchers have indicated that these signs may also be possible diagnostic indicators of a high cholesterol level.

For a complete analysis of the risks of obesity, and of being apple- or pear-shaped, see CC # 13.

RISK MULTIPLIES RISK

To obtain a true assessment of your heart disease risk, *all* risk factors must be considered, not merely your cholesterol components alone. Each additional risk factor multiplies the risk of all other factors. For example, a person with a total cholesterol level of 260 mgs/dl but no other risk factors, has a 17 per cent chance of experiencing a heart attack within the next ten years. But if that person also has severe hypertension, is 30 per cent overweight, and smokes three packs of cigarettes a day, that person's risk could be almost 100 per cent.

Since the risk attributable to each factor varies over a ten-fold range, and depends on the extent of all other risk factors, trying to assess your overall risk of having a heart attack could be a complicated task.

Fortunately, a software program called a Risk Factor Prediction Kit exists to estimate a person's overall chance of having a heart attack based on a combination of risk factors. Developed by the Framingham Heart Study, it rates your odds of having a heart attack based on your answers to questions about eight different risk factors.

If you have elevated cholesterol and one other risk factor, the computer might show that you are five times as likely to have a heart attack as a person with no risk factors. Almost all physicians today have this program. If you have any additional risk factors beyond high cholesterol, you can ask your doctor to include an overall Risk Factor Prediction when he evaluates your cholesterol test. Because the average American has a combination of risk factors, our national average chance of developing heart disease during a lifetime is 42 per cent.

Assuming elevated cholesterol is your only risk factor, having a total cholesterol as high as 300 mgs/dl may not be a cause for panic. With a level that high, the chances are good that, with the aid of the techniques in this book, you can easily drop it by 60 points in 60 days.

Alternatively, if your doctor's Risk Factor Prediction program finds that you have a combination of risks in addition to high cholesterol, then—with your doctor's permission—it could be imperative to begin using the full range of Cholesterol Cutter techniques in this book.

Fortunately, most other heart-disease risk factors can be lowered by the same techniques used for lowering cholesterol. So if you stay with them, the Cholesterol Cutters in this book can help to reverse almost every type of heart disease risk. They may even help to offset the effects of some genetic factors. Thousands of people with familial hypercholesterolemia have been able to cut their medications in half through upgrading their diet and lifestyle. Others have been able to get off drugs entirely.

HOW YOUR DOCTOR CAN GET YOU OFF DRUGS

Suppose you are already on drug treatment for high cholesterol. Should you replace cholesterol-lowering drugs you are already taking with a low-fat diet and other health-enhancing habits?

Assuming you are free of genetic risk factors, the answer is generally Yes—*but only with your doctor's full permission and cooperation*. If you are already taking a prescription drug, or an OTC drug, on your doctor's recommendation, or if you are under medical treatment for any reason at all, you must seek your doctor's approval and cooperation before reducing the dosage and phasing out the drug.

Generally, drugs prescribed for lowering cholesterol or for hypertension, heart disease, angina or artery spasm can be gradually reduced as an upgraded eating plan and a healthier lifestyle make them unnecessary. In this regard, we might mention that a physician practitioner of preventive medicine may be more willing to help you get off drugs than the typical M.D. So don't hesitate to seek a second opinion.

Doctors today are under tremendous pressure from pharmaceutical companies to place as many people as possible on lifelong maintenance drugs, such as those for lowering cholesterol or blood pressure. In fact, some medical writers have accused the pharmaceutical industry of pressuring the

NIH to launch its NCEP crusade in order to place as many Americans as possible on cholesterol-lowering drugs for life.

If you believe you are being kept on a drug you may not really need, seek a second medical opinion. Try to find a physician who believes that most drugs do only what a healthy body can do for itself.

NOT ALL DOCTORS ARE EQUALLY COMPETENT

Not all doctors are equally competent. Even within medicine, a choice of regimes exists for treating high cholesterol. A second doctor may be willing to use a preventive medicine approach that will allow you to replace drugs with some of the Cholesterol Cutters in this book. Be certain, however, to have a doctor's permission before you phase out any drugs you may be taking now.

And please bear in mind that the natural therapies in this book are for use only *after* your doctor has evaluated your full Heart Disease Risk Profile cholesterol test, and has given you clearance to make dietary changes, to eat more fiber, to begin an exercise program, and to undertake a stress management program as described in CCs # 16, 17 and 18.

Each person's heart disease risk must be assessed individually. Generally, this is how a doctor typically looks at elevated cholesterol.

If your total cholesterol is 240 mgs/dl or above; or if your total cholesterol is between 200-239 accompanied by up to two other risk factors; or if you already have some form of heart disease—then your doctor will look up your LDL level.

If your LDL is above 160mgs/dl., your physician should prescribe a low-fat diet and lifestyle program for a period of six months. Most mainstream physicians recommend the

AHA's Step One dietary plan (cut dietary fat to 30 per cent of calories or less; cut saturated fat to ten per cent of calories or less; and cut cholesterol to a maximum of 300 mgs daily). If this fails to lower your total cholesterol and LDL, your doctor may then prescribe the Step Two dietary plan (cut dietary fat to 25 per cent of calories or less; saturated fat to six or seven per cent or less; and cholesterol to a maximum of 200 mgs or less). If, after several more months, this also fails to lower your total cholesterol and LDL, your doctor may then prescribe drugs.

Your doctor would probably follow the same procedure if your LDL is above 130 mgs/dl and you have up to two other risk factors. Unless you have several risk factors, if your LDL is below 130 mgs/dl., you will normally be considered at relatively low risk.

HAVING SEVERAL MODERATE RISK FACTORS CAN BE DANGEROUS

Something your doctor may not be aware of are new studies showing that having three moderate risk factors may be actually more dangerous than having a single very high risk factor. For instance, having severe hypertension may not be as dangerous as having borderline-high blood pressure, mildly-elevated cholesterol and being moderately overweight.

New information from the Framingham Heart Study has shown that people with several slightly-elevated risk factors have a greater risk of heart disease than does a person with one single very high risk factor. Many doctors still may not recognize these dangers. And, in fact, many doctors are still unaware of the risk of having a triglycerides above 150 mgs/dl coupled with an HDL below 40.

CRITICISMS OF LOW CHOLESTEROL
SHOWN TO BE INVALID

How about studies that allegedly link a low cholesterol level with increased risk of stroke, or with increased risk of colon cancer?

A study of 350,977 men aged 35-57 by University of Minnesota researchers, and reported in the *New England Journal of Medicine* (April 6, 1989) found that while men with high cholesterol were at increased risk of stroke caused by blood clots, men with very low cholesterol levels had a three times greater risk than normal of a bleeding (hemorrhagic) stroke. This higher risk from bleeding strokes was limited to men with a total cholesterol below 160 mgs/dl *plus* hypertension (a diastolic blood pressure of 90 or higher).

Regardless of cholesterol level, *everyone* with high blood pressure is at greater risk for hemorrhagic stroke. However, if you have a total cholesterol of 170 or below, together with hypertension (a relatively rare combination), you should consult your doctor regarding the possibility of adding slightly more fat to your diet. A low total cholesterol may reduce the blood's ability to coagulate readily, and this could increase risk of a hemorrhagic stroke (while simultaneously reducing risk of a stroke or heart attack due to a blood clot). A slight increase in dietary fat might increase the blood's ability to coagulate and clot.

Nonetheless, the basic reason why people with high blood pressure have more strokes is because high blood pressure is a major risk factor for hemorrhagic stroke. Normotensive people with low cholesterol levels have no greater risk of hemorrhagic stroke than anyone else. The higher stroke rate in China, Japan and other Asian countries is due to hypertension resulting from widespread cigarette smoking and from the excessive use of salt.

Again, in some studies, a cholesterol level of 180 mgs/dl or below has appeared to be linked to higher incidence of colon cancer. However, extensive epidemiological studies of large populations in China, Japan and some Third World countries have proved the very opposite. The China Health Study and others have clearly demonstrated that nations which have the lowest average cholesterol levels also have the lowest cancer rates, not only for colon cancer but for most other cancers also.

A far more likely explanation is that having colon cancer leads to a lower cholesterol level. In the U.S., for example, both the Seventh Day Adventists and Mormons follow a low-fat diet and have lower average cholesterol levels than the general public. They also live five to seven years longer, while both men and women have a heart disease rate one-tenth that of the U.S. average, and a colon cancer rate barely half that of the U.S. general population. Thus the cholesterol-colon cancer link appears to be completely invalid.

Most objections to having a low cholesterol level appear to emanate from people who are desperately trying to find reasons why they should not upgrade their diet and lifestyle. Nonetheless, most doctors advise not allowing your total cholesterol to drop much below 120 mgs/dl.

BEYOND THE CHOLESTEROL HEADLINES

Once your cholesterol has stabilized at a satisfactorily low level, and you are staying with your cholesterol-lowering program, you should monitor your progress with a cholesterol test every three months.

New on the scene as this was written are do-it-yourself home cholesterol testers. Taking a sample of blood from capillaries in the fingertip, the device gives a readout of your total cholesterol in the form of a color gradation on a strip of paper. Current models take about 15 minutes to complete the test, each of which costs $10-$15. Despite lack of a printed readout, accuracy is within 5 per cent. The principal drawback appears to be use of blood from your finger, a factor already noted earlier in this chapter as a major cause of inaccurate readings. Although present home testers show only the total cholesterol, a home tester for HDL and triglycerides may appear soon.

After your cholesterol has remained satisfactorily low for one full year, you need check it again only once every five years. Naturally, this assumes that you stay with your cholesterol-lowering program. People who slip back into their former ways of eating and living invariably see their cholesterol shoot right back up. Just two weeks on a high-fat diet can send your total cholesterol soaring by 40 points or more.

Genetic factors excepted, we have almost total personal control over every risk factor for high cholesterol and heart disease. And we can easily modify these risks by using the Cholesterol Cutters in this book.

Which should remind us once more that cholesterol is merely one of a dozen risk factors, some of which may be more dangerous than cholesterol itself. Knowing this may give you a different perspective on just how scary a high cholesterol level really is.

CHAPTER THREE

Start Lowering Your Cholesterol Now

Provided you have already taken your full Heart Disease Risk Profile cholesterol test (see Chapter 2), you can start putting the principles below to work while you are reading the rest of this book.

Here are ten simple dietary changes that will really start your cholesterol heading down.

1. Cut out all organ meats, red meat and fatty luncheon meats and replace them with extra lean meat or, better, skinless chicken or turkey, or fish.

2. Eat not more than two whole eggs per week. However, you may eat additional egg whites provided you discard the yolks.

3. Keep butter or margarine use to one or two teaspoons a day or less.

4. Use only olive or canola oil for cooking or baking and keep their use to a minimum. Avoid all other fats and oils, including peanut butter and vegetable shortening.

5. Cut out all whole milk and low-fat dairy products and replace with skim milk or plain, non-fat yogurt.

6. Eliminate all regular commercial spreads, salad dressings, mayonnaise and sour cream, and replace with low-fat or non-fat versions.

7. Replace all baked goods, pies, cheesecakes, pastries, cookies, doughnuts, candy and chocolate with frozen non-fat desserts, pretzels, fig newtons, plain air-popped popcorn, or fresh fruit.

8. Cut out *all* fried foods and bake, steam, boil, broil or poach instead.

9. Replace all regular ice cream with plain, non-fat yogurt or with frozen non-fat dessert.

10. Replace all packaged, prepared, processed or manufactured convenience foods with fresh fruits, vegetables, whole grains and legumes.

Naturally, these are only suggestions. You may not want to adopt them all, nor be able to.

Nonetheless, these steps will get you started. But to really learn more about the low-cholesterol way to eat and live, you must read the rest of this book to the end.

CHAPTER FOUR

Unlocking the Secrets of Cholesterol Pathology

Increasing your knowledge is the first step in gaining power over your cholesterol. The more you know about the cholesterol process and how it threatens health, the less reason you have to fear cholesterol and heart disease.

Cholesterol itself is a soft, white, fatty sterol (alcohol) which exists only in foods of animal origin, that is in fish, flesh or fowl plus eggs and dairy products. Although its melting point is 300°F and it remains solid in the body, it is far from being toxic or poisonous. In our bodies, cholesterol plays an essential role in the formation of bile acids, various hormones, cell membranes, and in the conversion of sunlight to Vitamin D.

Cholesterol does not exist in the plant kingdom. Every fruit, vegetable, grain, nut, seed and legume is entirely free of cholesterol.

Since man appears to have evolved as a plant-eating primate, the human body was designed to synthesize its entire cholesterol needs from sources in plant foods. *We have no nutritional need for cholestrol in the diet at all.* Using nutrients in plant foods that we consume, the liver is completely capable of producing up to 1,500 mgs of cholesterol each day—more than enough to supply the body's every need.

The liver produces this cholesterol in response to the calory content of the food we consume. Since carbohydrates and protein each contain only four calories per gram, the liver produces only a moderate amount of cholesterol when we eat plant foods.

HOW FAT BOOSTS CHOLESTEROL LEVELS

By comparison, fat contains nine calories per gram. When we consume fat, and especially saturated fat, the liver more than doubles its cholesterol production.

Saturated fat, which occurs mostly in meat and dairy products (but also in some plant foods such as palm and coconut oils) provides an important source of nutrients from which the liver manufactures cholesterol. The result is that fat-rich foods like butter, red meat, cheese, ice cream and whole milk products are so high in saturated fats that, compared to most plant foods, they stimulate the liver to manufacture from one-and-half to three times as much cholesterol as normal, and often more.

To make it clearer, when we absorb ten mgs of dietary cholesterol, we merely add ten mgs of cholesterol into the bloodstream plus a small additional amount from the liver. But when we absorb ten mgs of saturated fat from the diet, the liver may respond by synthesizing 15-30 mgs or more of cholesterol. This surfeit of liver-produced cholesterol is then fed into the blood stream.

Foods of animal origin include all fish, seafood, eggs, fowl, meats and dairy products. Even extra-lean or low-fat animal foods have roughly 70 mgs of cholesterol per quarter pound. This dietary cholesterol that we consume in almost all food of animal origin is then added to the liver-produced cholesterol already in the blood stream.

CHOLESTEROL OVERDOSE

When we eat a plant-based diet, the liver produces cholesterol that is roughly equivalent to the body's needs. But when we consume a diet high in animal fats—primarily saturated fat and cholesterol—we quickly overload the body's ability to metabolize cholesterol. We create a surplus of cholesterol that, in the majority of Americans, ends up blocking the arteries and cutting off oxygen to the heart, brain and limbs.

In most people, the cholesterol levels revealed by the blood test are directly related to the amount of cholesterol deposits that exist in the arteries. The higher the total cholesterol and LDL levels, the more likely are the arteries to be blocked with cholesterol plaque—a condition known in medicine as atherosclerosis.

You don't need a degree in biochemistry to realize by now that the principal cause of high cholesterol is *saturated fat in the diet*. Culprit #2 is *cholesterol in the diet*. The conservative AHA recommends limiting dietary cholesterol to not more than 300 mgs per day. But the average American male

61

still consumes 435 mgs—135 mgs per day more than the AHA recommends (and 335mgs more than the preventive medicine recommendation).

Although the average American woman consumes only 304 mgs of cholesterol daily, virtually everyone in the U.S. above age two eats more saturated fat and cholesterol than their bodies can handle.

Culprit #3 is the *total amount of fat consumed in the diet*. The AHA recommends that not more than 30 per cent of calories be derived from fat while authorities in preventive medicine recommend that not more than ten per cent of calories should come from fat. In real life, however, almost 40 per cent of the average American's calories are still derived from fat. Although other types of fat like poly- and mono-unsaturated fats do not directly raise the cholesterol level, they still raise calorie and fat intake, thus contributing to obesity.

Saturated fat! Dietary cholesterol! Total fat intake! These three lipid factors are the direct causes of a high cholesterol level. They are also responsible for the accompanying risk of heart disease or stroke resulting from occlusion of the arteries by atherosclerosis.

However, cholesterol levels in the blood stream, and the extent of atherosclerosis, are strongly influenced by other counter-productive lifestyle habits. For example, cholesterol plaque tends to accumulate more rapidly at any place where an artery has been injured. Among principal causes of artery injury are smoking, hypertension, emotional stress, and free radicals emanating from poly-unsaturated fats in the diet.

LIPOPROTEINS—
THE CARRIERS OF CHOLESTEROL

Since cholesterol is soluble only in fat, it cannot flow through the water-based bloodstream by itself. It must be "ferried" inside a water-soluble bubble of protein. When the *protein* encapsulates the cholesterol (a *lipid*), it becomes a *lipoprotein*. Lipoproteins are produced in the liver in response to the demands caused by eating a high-fat meal. Lipoproteins are thus a form of cholesterol and there are five types in all.

Cholymicrons, the largest, appear in the intestinal walls several hours after digesting a fatty meal. They carry the fat and cholesterol just eaten through the bloodstream to the liver. En route, some of their triglycerides and cholesterol may be deposited in artery walls. Since cholymicrons disappear within ten hours of eating, they never register on a cholesterol test. Yet these ghost-like lipoproteins *can* deposit significant amounts of cholesterol into the arteries—one more reason why we should always eat a low-fat diet.

Once in the liver, both liver-produced and dietary cholesterol combine. The liver is also the receptacle for storing triglycerides (circulating blood fats) which it manufactures from carbohydrates, fatty acids, alcohol and cholesterol. Lipoprotein particles then transport these lipids through the blood stream to cells all over the body.

Roughly ten per cent of the cholesterol, and all of the triglycerides, are carried in VLDLs (Very Low Density Lipoproteins), the second largest lipoprotein. Some cholesterol also travels in IDLS (Intermediate Density Lipoproteins), third largest of the lipoproteins and a type that is seldom elevated and is therefore of little concern. But over 70 per cent of cholesterol is carried in LDLs (Low Density Lipoproteins), fourth largest of the lipoprotein particles.

The lower the density of the lipoprotein bubble, the more triglycerides and cholesterol it can carry. VLDLs and LDLs carry the bulk of the body's cholesterol through the blood stream to supply its billions of cells. They access body cells by traveling through the arteries and out into tiny tissue capillaries.

Here, body cells in need of triglycerides attract VLDLs by growing special receptors. As VLDL particles bind to these receptors, enzymes release the VLDL's triglycerides load into the cells. Almost immediately, the fat-depleted VLDL is transformed into an LDL.

Body cells in need of cholesterol also grow more LDL receptors on their outer walls. LDL particles, attracted to these receptors, bind on to them and disgorge their load of cholesterol into the cell.

OUR GENES CODE OUR CHOLESTEROL BASELINES

Over 20 human genes are involved in coding each person's baseline level of cholesterol metabolism. Each of us has an individual baseline level of LDL receptors in the liver. These are proteins on the surface of liver cells that remove LDL from the blood stream. When we eat saturated fat, it binds with LDL receptors in the liver, preventing these receptors from extracting LDLs from the blood stream. Through a variety of such mechanisms, saturated fat boosts our cholesterol levels to a far greater extent than does dietary cholesterol alone. For this reason, cutting saturated fat intake by five per cent will lower LDL and cholesterol levels approximately one-and-a-half to three times as much as will cutting dietary cholesterol by five per cent.

This doesn't mean that cholesterol is now safe to eat. It simply means that saturated fat is several times more dangerous.

Another genetic baseline controls the rate of cholesterol manufactured by the liver. Still another codes the baseline level of LDL receptors on each of our body cells.

Hence the body's rate of cholesterol production, and the speed at which LDL particles are removed from the blood stream, are both genetically influenced. And these levels vary considerably from one individual to another.

In 1985, Doctors Joseph Goldstein and Michael Brown were awarded a Nobel prize for the discovery of LDL receptors. They found that when body cells become satiated with cholesterol, the cells reduce their number of receptors. Satiation generally occurs when total cholesterol reaches 160 mgs/dl or more and LDL exceeds 90.

This leaves millions of cholesterol-loaded LDLs in the bloodstream with nowhere to go. In people who eat a diet high in fats and oils, free radicals may oxidize much of this surplus LDL. In the process, they set in motion an essential step in the formation of cholesterol plaque in artery walls.

HOW HDL CONQUERS CHOLESTEROL

HDLs (High Density Lipoproteins) are the smallest lipoprotein particles and they carry the smallest cholesterol load. Their task is to carry surplus cholesterol from tissue cells back to the liver where it is excreted. People who eat a plant-based diet generally have a total cholesterol below 160 mgs/

dl. At this low level, surplus cholesterol hardly exists. Thus the body's need for a high level of HDL is much lower than in meat-eating Americans.

By contrast, the average American on a high-fat diet produces large amounts of excess cholesterol. HDLs are the only way this surplus cholesterol can be carried from body cells back to the liver for excretion. Thus for people who eat the standard American diet, having a low HDL level can be dangerous.

The existence of HDL receptors on body cells is a recent discovery by biologist Jack Orem of the University of Washington. Dr. Orem found that when a cell becomes overloaded with cholesterol, it grows more HDL receptors on its surface. These attract and bind with HDL particles in the blood stream. When contact is made, enzymes shunt the cell's surplus cholesterol through the receptor into the HDL carrier.

Since our arteries are not mere rigid tubes but are living organisms, their walls are lined by living cells. HDL particles provide "reverse cholesterol transportation" to these cells by ferrying surplus cholesterol dumped there by LDLs back to the liver. In this way, HDLs actually cleanse the arteries.

THE DANGERS OF
GENETICALLY HIGH CHOLESTEROL

The baseline level of HDL receptors in our cells is genetically determined. Together, our baseline levels of LDL and HDL receptors determine our cholesterol metabolism.

These factors cause some people to have a genetic predisposition to high cholesterol and heart disease. Approximately five to ten per cent of the U.S. population is at risk for some degree of familial hypercholesterolemia. This, and associated diseases, can result in even young people having a total cholesterol as high as 1,000 mgs/dl and suffering a heart attack in their teens. Hypercholesterolemia is inability to remove cholesterol from the blood stream. Most people with a total cholesterol of 400 mgs/dl or more have some degree of hypercholesterolemia.

THE BENEFITS OF
GENETICALLY LOW CHOLESTEROL

Working in the opposite direction, these same genetic baselines can code for a high level of LDL receptors in the liver plus an equally high level of both LDL and HDL receptors on tissue cells. As a result, people with these fortunate genes are genetically endowed with a permanently low level of LDLs and a high level of HDLs. Regardless how much saturated fat and cholesterol they eat, only a moderate amount reaches the blood stream and any excess is swiftly removed by their high population of HDLs.

These people generally have a total cholesterol level of 160 mgs/dl or below, and they are virtually immune to coronary artery disease. A genetically-coded high level of LDL and HDL receptors may explain how Uncle George manages to put away three fried eggs, half a dozen sizzling strips of bacon, and a plateful of fries every morning and still live to be a healthy 93.

This may cause some people to ask if your total cholesterol level is low, can you safely eat a fat-rich diet with unlimited amounts of meat and cheese? If your total cholesterol stays

67

below 160 mgs/dl while you continue to eat the standard American diet, you may be one of these people. But in America, people whose cholesterol levels are not sensitive to dietary cholesterol and saturated fat are the exception. In most people, eating a diet high in saturated fat and cholesterol will raise both LDL and total cholesterol levels. And for every one per cent your total cholesterol level rises, your risk of heart disease increases by two per cent. Moreover, regardless of lipoprotein levels, a high fat diet is still a major risk factor for cancer, diabetes and other chronic diseases.

DIETARY CHOLESTEROL CAN STILL BE HAZARDOUS TO YOUR HEALTH

Furthermore, the work of Dr. Jeremiah Stamler of Northwestern University Medical School has demonstrated that, even though dietary cholesterol is now considered less dangerous than saturated fat, eating cholesterol-rich foods can still promote heart disease in people with a total cholesterol level as low as 175-200 mgs/dl.

A number of other studies have also suggested that dietary cholesterol has additional adverse effects on health over and above raising total cholesterol. These include increased risk of cancer, diabetes and obesity. One large study showed that a man of 46 who consumed three egg yolks a day cut four years from his life expectancy.

(To digress for a moment: not all studies have cast eggs as the villain. While eggs are probably the highest single source of dietary cholesterol (213 mgs per egg yolk), they are comparatively low in saturated fat (1.7 grams per yolk). This may explain why some studies have shown that excessive egg

68

consumption elevates serum cholesterol while others have concluded that eggs have little effect in raising a person's total cholesterol. Nonetheless, we might add that eggs are still high in animal protein which some researchers have identified as contributing to cancer and to renal and heart disease. Eggs also contribute nothing in the way of dietary fiber.)

A healthy heart pumps four to five quarts of blood per minute through the arteries and it can continue to pump efficiently, without weakening, for well over a century. To do so, however, it requires an abundant supply of oxygen-laden blood.

Feeding the heart muscle with this vital oxygen are the coronary arteries, a network of blood vessels that radiate down over the top of the heart and encircle it. Each artery is approximately .1 - .2 inches in diameter. When healthy, these arteries are clean, wide, elastic, flexible and smooth on the inner surface.

THE MULTIPLE CAUSES OF ARTERY INJURY

Unfortunately, most Americans eat a diet and follow a lifestyle that exposes their bodies to dietary, emotional and environmental stresses. The coronary arteries, and all others, can be injured or damaged by stresses arising from:

1. Carbon monoxide toxins from smoking.
2. The pounding pressure of hypertension.
3. Free radicals arising from the oxidization of LDL cholesterol.
4. A high level of total cholesterol and LDL cholesterol in the blood stream.

5. Poor muscle tone arising from lack of exercise.
6. A surfeit of animal protein and fat in the diet.
7. Excessive amounts of salt in the diet.
8. Toxins from stress hormones in the blood stream.

The inner walls of arteries are lined by special endothelium cells. Their role is to prevent clots by sensing and responding to changes in blood flow. It is in these cells that one, or a combination of the stresses just discussed, can initiate an injury.

Endothelium cells may also be damaged by dietary methionine. This amino acid is abundant in animal fat and protein. Once in the body it turns into homocysteine which directly damages endothelium cells.

According to Louis Tobias, M.D., professor of medicine at the University of Minnesota Hospital in Minneapolis, excessive amounts of dietary salt can also cause artery damage independent of its possible action in creating high blood pressure.

Pounding by blood under abnormally high pressure at bends in arteries is a common cause of endothelium cell damage in people with hypertension. And toxins in cigarette smoke are one of the *primary* causes of artery damage.

Lack of physical exercise can also cause loss of muscle tone throughout the body, including the tone of the smooth muscles which surround each artery. This loss of muscle tone can lead to an abnormal and often injurious cell biology in the endothelium cells that line each artery's inner surface.

A high cholesterol level in the blood stream may also irritate endothelium cells. Whenever total cholesterol is above 160 mgs/dl and LDL above 100, some degree of irritation and eventual injury may be caused to these cells.

Further irritation to artery walls is caused by the presence

70

of stress hormones released into the blood stream when we experience negative emotions like anger, hate, hostility or fear.

Risk of injury is also accelerated by advancing age and by the total number of heart disease risk factors. Diabetes also intensifies all forms of arterial injury.

In non-smokers, a major source of artery damage are the free radicals released from fats in the bloodstream.

HOW FREE RADICALS
CREATE CHOLESTEROL PLAQUE

Based on very recent discoveries, a growing number of researchers are convinced that, without the role played by free radicals, cholesterol blockage could not exist.

A free radical is a molecular fragment that has an unpaired electron. Highly reactive, these free radicals search to regain a full complement of electrons. Whenever LDL particles are exposed to these unstable molecules, the result is to oxidize each LDL particle. Immediately, the LDL becomes stickier, a quality which increases risk of platelet clumping and formation of a blood clot. In the process, an oxidized LDL particle becomes toxic to the human body.

This fact is immediately recognized by patrolling macrophage cells. Charged with defending the body against invading toxins, these "soldier" cells of the immune system constantly patrol the arteries on a search-and-destroy mission.

Essentially, a macrophage is a scavenger cell that engulfs and swallows every toxic particle it finds. Whenever a macrophage encounters oxidized LDLs, it consumes them. The arteries of people who eat a high-fat diet are frequently lined by macrophages bloated with oxidized LDL particles.

71

Creating artery blockage involves an amazingly complex interplay of different body mechanisms. For example, injured areas in artery walls exude molecules of Platelet Derived Growth Factor. This substance lures macrophages loaded with oxidized LDLs through the injured surface of artery walls and into the artery wall itself. As a layer of endothelial cells grows back over the injury, the macrophage, along with its load of LDL cholesterol, is permanently trapped inside the artery wall.

Very possibly, dozens or hundreds of LDL-loaded macrophages are trapped in a single injured spot. There, imbedded macrophages bulge out into the arterial wall.

This initial stage in atherosclerosis appears as a fatty, yellow stripe or streak on the walls of the body's larger arteries. Yellow streaks of atherosclerosis are plainly visible on the arteries of at least half of all American pre- and adolescent boys. The extent of these yellow streaks corresponds almost exactly with the amount of animal fat and whole milk dairy foods in each youngster's diet.

With the passing of time, these lesions protrude into the bloodstream and become traps for passing debris. Each lesion ensnares a collection of triglycerides, collagen, fibrin (a clotting agent), sticky blood platelets and dead cells. Over the years, the mass forms a hard deposit known as atheromatous plaque.

Calcium then coats it, forming a rough surface where still more debris collects. Gradually, as the years pass, and a high-fat diet continues to be eaten, the plaque grows relentlessly larger. Eventually, it protrudes out into the artery, causing the artery to narrow or occlude and to seriously impede blood flow.

72

THE FREE RADICAL THEORY OF CHOLESTEROL

Free radicals generally occur only in oils and fats and in fatty foods of animal origin. Food fried in oils and fats abound in free radicals. The forced feeding and growth hormones used to fatten cattle in feedlots make red meat another concentrated source of free radicals. Just about all foods high in fat and cholesterol—especially polyunsaturated vegetable oils—are potentially high sources of free radicals.

By contrast, many plant-based foods are rich in anti-oxidants, each capable of neutralizing one or more free radicals. A diet high in whole grains, fruits and vegetables is the richest dietary source of anti-oxidants.

A diet of plant-based foods provides double protection from heart disease. First, because fruits, vegetables and whole grains contain very few free radicals to begin with. And second, they are rich in anti-oxidants which can knock out any free radicals that do happen to stray into the arteries.

Specifically, the most powerful anti-oxidants found in plant foods are Vitamins C and E, beta-carotene and selenium. Several large population studies have already shown that people who consume plant foods rich in these nutrients are many times less likely to suffer from heart disease, stroke, cancer and other common degenerative diseases than the general public.

Perhaps the following idea has already crossed your mind. Since anti-oxidants appear capable of preventing the formation of cholesterol plaque, could you safeguard yourself against heart disease risk by taking anti-oxidants in supplement form while you continue to eat a high-fat diet?

Sorry! But sprinkling Vitamins C and E on your ham and eggs won't do the trick. What the free radical theory of cholesterol does is to emphasize the double protective

73

whammy provided by a plant-based diet. First, plant foods release very few, if any, of the free radicals needed to create blockage. Second, most plant foods are loaded with anti-oxidants that destroy free radicals.

Could you ask for a better deal? For more details, turn to CC#14 and learn how to protect your arteries from free radical damage the natural way.

ARTERIAL BLOCKS ARE THE CAUSE OF MOST CARDIOVASCULAR DISEASE

To some extent, atherosclerosis occurs in arteries throughout the body. But it is in the coronary and carotid arteries, and in arteries in the legs, where the effect is most severe. Atherosclerosis in the coronary arteries can cause angina or a heart attack. Atherosclerosis in the carotid arteries located in the neck, can choke off the blood supply to the brain, creating cerebral vascular disease or stroke. And atherosclerosis in arteries in the legs can cause peripheral vascular disease or claudication, an excruciating pain which makes walking impossible and can lead to gangrene and amputation.

Occlusion of smaller blood vessels can also lead to congestive heart failure, eye disease or kidney failure. Cholesterol blockage of penile arteries is also a common cause of impotence in men over fifty. In each case, high cholesterol levels are the underlying cause. Without an excess of cholesterol, atherosclerosis can scarcely exist.

Efforts by Americans to stop smoking, to cut fat consumption and to increase exercise have significantly reduced the incidence of cardiovascular disease. But the average American still has one chance in two of dying from a cholesterol-related disease.

Each year, one-and-a-half million Americans—half under age 65—still have a heart attack and 511,000 die. Of those who survive, 24 per cent are left with reduced physical ability and 11 per cent are incapacitated. Another 500,000 Americans suffer strokes each year. Of the survivors, 66 per cent are physically impaired.

The underlying cause of almost all this death and disablement is high cholesterol levels provoked by dietary fat, smoking, unresolved emotional stress and a sedentary lifestyle.

ARTERY BLOCKAGE BEGINS IN INFANCY

According to two major studies of American youngsters—the 18-year Bogalusa study of 8,000 Louisiana children, and the NIH-funded P-Day study (Pathological Determinant of Atherosclerosis in Youth)—atheroclerosis begins in infancy, and, in most people, progresses throughout life.

Starting at age 10-12, fatty streaks appear in the arteries of at least 50 per cent of young males. By age 19-21, these streaks have become fibrous plaque and are already restricting arterial blood flow. By age 33, the plaques have become lesions and are blocking up to 40 per cent of the diameter of the coronary arteries. By age 44, calcification has coated both the lesions and arterial walls with a hard covering of calcium. Lesions are now large, scarred and potentially occlusive.

Before reaching age 65, one-third of all Americans have a heart attack, stroke or claudication. And after 65, the rate increases.

Few symptoms are noticed until the coronary arteries are 50 per cent blocked. At this point, angina is likely. Upon exertion, a pressure, heaviness or pain in the chest will occur and it may radiate into the neck, left arm or shoulder or even into the teeth. After resting one to three minutes, angina pain due to exertion usually disappears. But it is a solemn reminder that the coronary arteries are severely blocked and that a heart attack could occur at any time.

NEGATIVE EMOTIONS TRIGGER MOST HEART ATTACKS

Millions of Americans aged 50 and over—those who continue to eat the standard American diet—typically have a 50 per cent blockage in one coronary artery and a 65 per cent blockage in another. Amazingly, a sedentary person can still function on these blockages.

But if angry thoughts trigger rage, hostility or cynicism, they can set off the "fight or flight" response. This is a hair trigger reaction that prepares the body to meet imminent physical danger. The sympathetic nervous system, the emergency branch of the autonomic nervous system, takes over and all systems are GO. The adrenal glands squirt hormones into the bloodstream to speed up body functions. Nerve fibers signal the smooth muscles to constrict every artery, including the coronary and carotid arteries, and those in the legs. Blood pressure shoots up. And the clogging ability of blood platelets rises to prevent bleeding in case of a possible wound.

The effect of this response on arteries already partially occluded by atherosclerosis can be devastating. First, that portion of the artery still left open is now half-closed by constriction of the smooth muscle. Secondly, platelets in the blood stream become sticky and clump into a clot. It takes just one of these tiny clots to completely block blood flow through the already constricted and occluded artery.

HOW BLOOD CLOTS CAUSE HEART ATTACKS

Many cardiologists now believe that the majority of heart attacks are caused by blood clots that result from a fit of rage, anxiety, hostility or biting sarcasm. Several studies have shown that these stressful emotions can also raise cholesterol levels.

Sudden blockage of an already occluded artery can create a coronary insufficiency, causing portions of the heart muscle to be deprived of oxygen and to turn blue and die. All this is usually accompanied by tremendous pressure or pain in the chest, neck and jaw, inside the left arm and shoulder, and between the shoulder blades. The pain may be continuous or spasmodic. Yet it differs from angina in that it lasts for two minutes or more and it cannot be relieved by nitroglycerine.

Accompanying symptoms often include shortness of breath, sweating, weakness, dizziness, nausea, vomiting or anxiety. Sometimes, however, there is a feeling of restlessness, apprehension or foreboding—the symptoms of a silent heart attack.

In either case, the sooner one can be taken to an intensive care unit, the better. Today, medications and hi-tech treatment can save the majority of heart attack victims who make it to the hospital on time. But it's not most peoples' idea of a fun trip.

THE TRAUMA OF SURGERY

If you have multi-vessel blockage, your doctor may still suggest a bypass operation. That means slicing your chest in half and prizing your ribs apart while your blocked coronary arteries are replaced with a vein stripped from your leg or chest. Currently, 368,000 bypass operations are still being performed annually despite sound evidence that a large percentage could have been treated just as successfully with drugs. One problem is that within ten years, approximately half of all vein bypasses have to be replaced a second time.

Or possibly your doctor may recommend an angioplasty in which a balloon catheter is threaded through blood vessels into the partially-blocked coronary artery. The balloon is then inflated to expand and unblock the artery. Here again, due to a condition called restinosis, about 30 per cent of arteries close again within a few months. Despite new laser catheters designed to minimize restinosis, the mortality risk may run as high as two per cent.

A similar operation called coronary atherectomy catheter uses a high-speed drill to open blocked arteries. But some cardiologists have suggested that any type of catheter surgery may actually accelerate atherosclerosis by causing minor injuries to artery walls.

Nowadays, as word of preventive medicine spreads, recovery by natural means without drugs or surgery is becoming an increasingly popular option for many. Yet millions of Americans are unable and unwilling to take an active role in their own recovery. For these unfortunate people, drugs or surgery remain the only choice.

HIGH CHOLESTEROL IS
THE CAUSE OF MOST STROKES

A stroke occurs when one of the carotid arteries is completely blocked. Part of the brain is then deprived of oxygen and a portion may die. Depending on location, you could lose your ability to speak, to hear, to see or to swallow. Or you could be paralyzed on one side.

In people with a total cholesterol above 180-200 mgs/dl., the carotid arteries can readily be blocked by atherosclerotic plaque. One reason is because the arteries narrow in the neck region and branch off into the internal and external carotids. This physiology makes carotid artery walls extremely vulnerable to injury. The internal carotids supply the brain, retina and optic nerve as well as brain areas at the base of the skull.

Most cases of stroke are actually triggered by blood clots just as are most heart attacks. They frequently occur at night or in the early morning when blood pressure is low.

HORMONES SAFEGUARD MOST YOUNGER WOMEN FROM HEART DISEASE

Most of the heart disease risk factors we've discussed so far have applied primarily to men. Until menopause, women's sex hormone, estrogen, boosts their HDL level and protects them from heart disease. However, cigarette smoking or diabetes can erode the protection of this hormone shield. Thus it is imperative for women of all ages to cease smoking and to maintain weight at the desirable level.

A good general rule is that women's risk of heart disease lags that of men by approximately one decade. A woman of 60 has about the same heart disease risk as a man of 50.

This doesn't mean that high cholesterol is a man's dysfunction. Six times as many women die each year from heart disease as from breast cancer. One reason is that women have smaller arteries than men, making them easier for atherosclerosis to block. Women also tend to have higher triglycerides, a condition often accompanied by an increase in total and LDL cholesterol levels.

Once past menopause, a woman's heart disease risk gradually rises to equal that of men. Total cholesterol and LDL levels skyrocket in women who continue to eat the standard American diet. More than half of all women over 65 have high blood pressure. Almost 40 per cent of older women who have heart attacks are obese. And by age 65, heart disease is the major killer of American women.

The good news is that none of this needs to happen. By following our Chol-Tamer or Blockbuster Plans, women can lower their cholesterol levels as readily as men. Whether male or female, by keeping your total cholesterol below 160 mgs/dl and your LDL below 100—and provided you don't smoke or have diabetes—your heart disease risk can be minimal. The China Health Study also revealed that younger women who have a low cholesterol level also have a much lower risk of breast or colon cancer or diabetes.

LIFELONG BENEFITS OF LOW CHOLESTEROL

Cutting risk of heart disease and stroke isn't the only benefit of having low cholesterol. Study after study is finding that—in both men and women—the higher your cholesterol, the greater your risk for most cancers, Type II diabetes, renal disease and even osteoporosis and Alzheimer's Disease.

That's because *all* degenerative diseases—not merely heart disease and stroke—are caused by the same set of health-destroying lifestyle habits. Scores of major studies are now implicating animal fat and protein, overeating, lack of exercise, excess body weight, unresolved emotional stress and substance abuse as the underlying cause of *all* degenerative disease.

Experts at the National Cancer Institute believe that 75 per cent of all cancers arise from the standard American diet and our sedentary lifestyle and smoking habits. A ten year study of 448 men and women aged 75-85 at the Albert Einstein College of Medicine in New York City recently concluded that women who had a history of heart disease before entering the study were five times as likely to develop Alzheimer's, or other forms of dementia, by the study's end.

Another 1989 study by Dr. Jeremiah Stamler of Northwestern University Medical School showed that the higher a person's total cholesterol, the greater chance of developing cancer, diabetes and other chronic diseases. Meanwhile, Framingham Heart Study researchers report that people who eat the most cholesterol have the highest death rate from *all* causes, not merely from heart disease and stroke.

By adopting the Cholesterol Cutter techniques in this book, you can slash your risk of *all* killer diseases that arise from our affluent diet and lifestyle.

CHAPTER FIVE

How to Use
This Book

What cholesterol-lowering strategy should you adopt? Which of the 18 natural Cholesterol Cutter techniques should you use? And how far should you go into each one?

The answer depends on how low you wish your cholesterol to drop. Don't be surprised if your mainstream medical doctor has never heard of Dr. Dean Ornish or the China Health Study. Most physicians are too busy to stay abreast of the many new and exciting studies emerging from the leading edge of cholesterol research. Hence you may be told that if your total cholesterol is 199 mgs/dl or below, you are "safe."

By presenting information from other than mainstream sources, we believe we have given you facts so complete that you can draw your own conclusions. For instance, you can choose to settle for a "desirable" total cholesterol of 199 mgs/dl or below; you can choose to aim for a safe level of 180 or below; or you can aim for the ultimate security provided by a level of 160 or below.

Which level you decide to aim for depends on whose studies you believe in; and on how far you're willing to go in upgrading your lifestyle. As a result, this book doesn't advise any rigid cholesterol-lowering regime. In fact, after reading this book through, few people should have any difficulty in deciding on their own personal cholesterol-lowering strategy. And most of us will know instinctively which of the 18 Cholesterol Cutters we should incorporate into our plan.

Nonetheless, as a broad, general guide, we are suggesting three different, and purely optional, cholesterol-lowering plans. You can choose the one that most closely targets the cholesterol level you believe you should aim for. The plan you select should also be one with which you feel comfortable.

Here are the three basic plans.

TOTAL CHOLESTEROL TARGET, 199 MGS/DL OR BELOW: THE EASY-DOES-IT-PLAN

Similar to the AHA's Step One Formula, this lenient plan is based on the 55-30-15 way of eating. Translated, this means that at least 55 per cent of dietary calories are supplied by complex-carbohydrates (fresh, unprocessed fruits, vegetables, whole grains, legumes, seeds and nuts); a maximum of 30 per cent is from fat (of which not more than ten per cent is saturated, nor more than ten per cent polyunsaturated); and a maximum of 15 per cent is from protein.

The protein can include up to six ounces of very lean meat, fish or poultry each day, of which not more than three ounces consists of meat. If desired, an equivalent amount of plain, nonfat yogurt, skim milk or up to three egg whites may be substituted for all or part of the flesh food.

Cholesterol intake is limited to 100 mgs per 1,000 calories with a maximum of 300 mgs per day. Caffeine intake is restricted to two five-ounce cups of coffee per day. And smoking must cease.

Exercise should consist of gradually working up to a brisk walk of at least 20 minutes three or more times each week (see CC #12 for details).

For most Americans, following the Easy-Does-It Plan means reducing fat intake by about one fourth. In practice, this may not be enough to lower your total cholesterol by 30 points in 30 days. And it is too small a reduction to have much effect on lowering triglycerides.

Some cardiologists believe the recommendations are mainly cosmetic and that fat intake is still too high to take cholesterol down to really safe levels. Several writers have also suggested that the recommendations were watered down to satisfy the meat, egg and dairy industries. Nonetheless, given enough time, your total cholesterol should gradually drop to between 180-199 mgs/dl.

To put the Easy-Does-It Plan into practice, you need to have read and absorbed the contents of this book so far. We then recommend incorporating CCs # 1, 2, 3, 4, 5, 6, 7, 8, 9, 10, 11, 12 and 16 into your program.

TOTAL CHOLESTEROL TARGET, 180 MGS/DL OR BELOW: THE CHOL-TAMER PLAN

Based on AHA's Step Two formula, and the Ideal Diet recommended by the NAS, the Chol-Tamer (or Cholesterol-

Tamer) Plan, should effectively lower the average person's elevated cholesterol by 30 points in 30 days, with an eventual target level of 180 mgs/dl or below.

The eating plan breaks down into a 65-20-15 formula, meaning that 65 per cent of calories is provided by complex carbohydrates; a maximum of 20 per cent is derived from fat (with not more than six per cent from unsaturated fat, nor more than 7 per cent from polyunsaturated fat); and 15 per cent or less is from protein, a substantial portion of which is from plant-based sources.

The Plan allows three-and-one-half ounces daily of fish or skinless poultry or an equivalent amount of plain, nonfat yogurt or skim milk, or up to three egg whites daily. Smoking is forbidden while caffeine should be limited to one five-ounce cup of coffee per day.

Exercise should consist of gradually working up to a brisk walk of at least 25 minutes five times each week (see CC #12 for details).

To put the Chol-Tamer Plan into practice, you need to have read and absorbed the contents of this book so far. We then recommend incorporating CCs # 1, 2, 3, 4, 5, 6, 7, 8, 9, 10, 11, 12, 15, 16, and 17 into your program.

TOTAL CHOLESTEROL TARGET, 160 MGS/DL OR BELOW: THE BLOCKBUSTER PLAN

By incorporating all of the Cholesterol Cutters into one single program, the Blockbuster Plan should lower all but the most stubborn cholesterol levels by at least 30 points in 30 days. The Blockbuster Plan then aims to minimize the risk of cardiovascular disease by taking your total cholesterol down to the 150-160 mgs/dl range or below.

While your cholesterol level should plunge during the first few weeks, it may take several months to reach a totally safe level. By keeping your total cholesterol below 160 mgs/dl, the Blockbuster Plan also minimizes further risk of injury to arteries. Animal studies also suggest that by maintaining the total cholesterol level this low, endothelial function tends to recover, and the arteries begin to behave normally once more. The Blockbuster Plan is based, in part, on studies by the NIH's National Education Panel which has recommended the ideal cholesterol level as 150-160 mgs/dl; on research by the Framingham Heart Study, demonstrating that heart disease risk begins when the total cholesterol starts to rise above the 150-160 range; on findings by the Pritikin Program and Lifestyle Heart Trial; on the China Health Study; and on many other studies and recommendations in the field of preventive medicine.

Based on the 75-10-15 formula, the Blockbuster eating plan derives 75 per cent or more of its calories from complex-carbohydrates; up to ten per cent of calories from fat (with not more than two-and-one-half per cent from saturated fat, nor more than three per cent from poly-unsaturated fat); and up to 15 per cent of calories from protein, most of which is from plant sources.

Animal-derived foods are limited to one eight-ounce cup of plain, nonfat yogurt or skim milk, or up to three egg whites per day. This program automatically cuts fat to one-fourth that of the standard American diet while raising fiber intake to 25-35 grams daily. It also increases intake of most essential nutrients. The American Dietetic Association has confirmed that a primarily plant-based diet, such as this, meets all nutritional needs.

Smoking is unthinkable on the Blockbuster Plan while caffeine is totally eliminated.

Exercise consists of gradually working up to where you are walking briskly in your target heart range for 30 minutes or more five times a week. On two other days each week, you enjoy a longer 45-60 minute (or more) walk, preferably with a few hills along the way.

To put the Blockbuster Plan into practice, you need to have read and absorbed the contents of this book so far. We then recommend incorporating CCs # 1, 2, 3, 4, 5, 6, 7, 8, 9, 10, 11, 12, 15, 16, 17 and 18 into your program.

OTHER HELPFUL CHOLESTEROL CUTTERS

Not mentioned so far is CC #13: Lowering Cholesterol by Losing Belly Fat, which is primarily of interest only to those who are overweight, or who have a recognizable spare tire around the middle. If you are in this category, CC #13 is essential reading.

Also left to your discretion is CC #14: Nutrients That May Help Lower Cholesterol, which lists heart-protecting foods high in anti-oxidants and also describes nutritional supplements that provide strong support for most other Cholesterol Cutters. Specific guidelines concerning each of the three cholesterol-lowering plans is also given under CCs # 2, 3, 4, 5, 6, 12 and 15.

If you are tailoring your own personal cholesterol-lowering plan, to be effective, it must include CCs # 2, 3, 4, 6, 7, 8, 9, 10, 11 and 12 (plus 13 if you are overweight or apple-shaped).

INTERVENING IN AND FINE-TUNING YOUR CHOLESTEROL COMPONENTS

You can modify and fine-tune your LDL, HDL and VLDL cholesterol components, and also your triglycerides, by using one, or a combination, of Cholesterol Cutters.

To lower LDL, VLDL or triglycerides, for example, consider using CCs # 2, 3, 4, 6, 7, 8, 10, 11 and 13.

To raise your HDL level, look up CCs #12 and 13.

If triglycerides are a problem, look up CCs # 2, 4, 6, 11, 12, and 13.

To reduce stress, the underlying cause of many cases of high cholesterol, look up CCs # 15, 16, 17 and 18.

The actual CCs you select, and the extent to which you use them, will depend on how you choose to fine-tune and manipulate your cholesterol components.

None of the three cholesterol-lowering plans places any limit on calories. Provided you stay within the guidelines for fat and animal protein, you can eat unlimited quantities of food. And there are no limits on healthy snacks.

A REALISTIC GAME PLAN FOR LIFE

You will also quickly discover that these are not mere diets but a whole new eating plan for life. And we mean *for life*. If you go back to your former ways of eating and living, your cholesterol may very well go soaring back up.

The 30 points in 30 days claim is based on using the full eating recommendations of the plan you select from the very first day. For example, if you adopt only half the eating recommendations of the Chol-Tamer Plan, you will probably not lower your cholesterol by 30 points in 30 days. You must be following the eating recommendations *totally* from Day One. And you must have made at least a start on the exercise program.

If you prefer to get into things more gradually, consider adopting the Easy-Does-It Plan until your cholesterol has stabilized at a lower level. Then switch to the Chol-Tamer Plan until your cholesterol has stabilized at a still lower level. You can then continue to lower your cholesterol by embarking on the Blockbuster Plan.

Nonetheless, from several cardiac rehabilitation centers and cholesterol clinics comes word that many patients find it easier and simpler to go all the way into a program, such as the Chol-Tamer or Blockbuster Plan, than to ease in gradually by making partial changes.

KEEP YOUR APPROACH HOLISTIC

Whatever you do, try to keep your approach holistic by focusing equally on diet, exercise and stress management. Since know-how is the key to practicing holistic health, you must become a medically-informed layperson by reading and absorbing this book all the way through. You should then try to use as many different approaches as possible. Thus we urge you to read, and to use Cholesterol Cutters, from each of these chapters.

Chapter 6. The Motivational Approach.

Chapter 7. The Dietary Approach.

Chapter 8. The Physical Approach.

Chapter 9. The Nutritional Approach.

Chapter 10. The Stress Management Approach.

The more diversified the approaches you select, the more

89

holistic—and the more effective—your cholesterol-lowering program will be.

QUICK FIX FOR CHOLESTEROL

Don't worry about your cholesterol level falling too quickly. Losing cholesterol has no parallel with weight loss, in which rapid loss of weight can cause your weight to bounce back up again. No risk at all is involved in dropping your cholesterol by 40 points in 20 days. And for as long as you continue to follow our Cholesterol Cutters, your cholesterol level should remain gratifyingly low.

That about sums it up. By having read this far, you're already well on your way to a healthier heart and arteries. And the only side effects you're likely to experience are feeling better, healthier and younger, and reducing weight and stress.

CHAPTER SIX

The Motivational Approach

For most people, the biggest hurdle in lowering their cholesterol is not in learning how to do it, but in psyching themselves up to actually begin.

CHOLESTEROL CUTTER # 1:

HOW TO BECOME A WINNER AT THE CHOLESTEROL-LOWERING GAME

It can be quite a jolt to discover that we have high cholesterol and are at risk for a heart attack. But it could also be a powerful catalyst for changing the way we eat, live and think. It could force us to ask ourselves just where health ranks on our value scale.

We might ask, for example, whether continuing to live a high-fat, high-stress, and high-cholesterol lifestyle is worth a grieving spouse. Or would we prefer to spend 15 or 20 more years with our mate, and live to see our grandchildren grow up?

The picture we're given by the medical profession, and by the media, is that Americans are so weak and self-indulgent that it is hopeless to expect the majority to ever display the degree of self-discipline required to improve their diet or lifestyle.

Sure, we all want to lower our cholesterol—but without giving up our rich, high-fat food or having to exercise or to learn to handle stress. As a result, we are told, most Americans are just sitting out the cholesterol-lowering crusade, willing to take their chances.

Certainly this image is not without foundation. Millions of Americans have already chosen to die prematurely rather than to make the necessary lifestyle changes that science has shown could have made them virtually immune to heart attack and other killer diseases.

SUCCESS IS THE BEST MOTIVATOR

Yet this scenario overlooks one vital factor in the field of motivational psychology. Studies in this field have clearly demonstrated, time and again, that most people *are* willing to change their diet and lifestyle as long as they can begin to feel better within just a few days.

In other words, to become a winner at the cholesterol-lowering game, we need almost instant positive feedback.

Luckily, positive feedback in the form of feeling better swiftly is exactly what you are likely to experience by adopting our Chol-Tamer or Blockbuster Plans. These plans are almost identical to those that have been used for years at some of the most successful cholesterol-lowering clinics in the nation. Records show that virtually everyone who has adopted and adhered to one or the other of these plans has experienced almost immediate benefits to their health.

Within a week, literally hundreds of people have reported feeling better than they have in years. Almost all have reported losing several pounds as well as experiencing renewed energy and vigor, a strongly positive attitude, and soaring self-esteem. In fact, the benefits of their diet and lifestyle changes have been so overwhelming that any sacrifice has seemed insignificant by comparison.

Clearly, success is the best of all possible motivators. For example, under medical supervision, the Pritikin Program has achieved thousands of cases of dramatic improvement and recovery from almost every form of cardiovascular disease.

As far back as 1976, for example, out of 893 patients who attended the first 26-day Pritikin Program sessions, the overall rate of reduction in cholesterol and triglycerides levels was 25 per cent. Overweight patients lost, on average, 13 pounds per person. Sixty-two per cent of those taking drugs for angina were able to stop. Eighty-five per cent of hypertensive patients who were taking medication lowered their blood pressure to the point where drugs became unnecessary. And over half of those taking insulin for adult-onset diabetes no longer needed it. But the most astounding success concerned 64 patients who had been recommended by their doctors for bypass surgery. After five years on the Pritikin Program, 51 still did not require surgery.

SWIFT HEALTH BENEFITS

Tens of thousands of cases of similar health benefits—many apparent in as short a time as one week—have also been documented at the many cardiac rehabilitation centers across the country. During Dr. Dean Ornish's Lifestyle Heart Trial, for instance, 91 per cent of participants experienced a significant reduction in chest pain, usually within just a few weeks.

The literature is filled with cases of patients who, unable to walk across the room without chest pain, found themselves able to walk several miles after a few weeks on a combined low-fat diet and exercise program.

Naturally, all these benefits occurred during medically-supervised programs. And we make no claim that anyone following any of our three cholesterol-lowering plans will overcome any disease or dysfunction beyond lowering their cholesterol. Nonetheless, these medically-confirmed records do provide documented proof of the amazing health benefits that have occurred in a relatively short time when natural Cholesterol Cutter techniques were used to lower cholesterol and other risk factors for heart disease.

POSITIVE FEEDBACK BOOSTS MOTIVATION

For anyone who throws themselves wholeheartedly into either the Chol-Tamer or Blockbuster Plans, positive feedback should appear in just a few days. So plan to keep a daily written record of your progress. Note down how much less fat you are eating and how many more vegetables, fruits and whole grains. Keep a record of the distance you walk

94

each day, and of your weight and your resting pulse rate, and of how much better you feel with each passing day.

Each day you'll be encouraged by seeing your progress on paper. And you'll be constantly reminded of the benefits of lowering cholesterol naturally.

Most books about lowering cholesterol seem to assume that the average American is a weak-willed person who wavers easily, yields to every temptation, and would rather watch TV than walk up a hill.

Fortunately, we don't buy into this stereotyped image. To begin with, over 30 million Americans have quit smoking in recent years, an accomplishment several times more difficult than adopting any of the lifestyle changes needed to lower cholesterol. Moreover, studies are making it increasingly clear that our power to change is far greater than most of us think.

Many behavioral psychologists are saying that the only thing that really holds us back is our desire to remain in our "comfort zone." In response to the stress of growing up, we tend to create a comfortable lifestyle built around eating sweet and fatty foods, watching TV, and avoiding most forms of physical exertion. Collectively, these indulgences form our comfort zone. As some of us grow up, we call it the "Good Life."

Eating itself is a nurturing and comforting social act. Most of us continue to eat what we ate as we grew up, a learned behavior that becomes a deeply ingrained part of our culture. As we reach adulthood, eating fat continues to be comforting because it reinforces memories of when we were given these same foods to comfort us as youngsters.

As we become older, we continue to rely on rich, fatty foods to comfort us and to tranquilize us against the stress of daily living. By the time we're in our 20s, we so crave being in the comfort zone that the majority of us assume we are locked into these habits for life.

GETTING OUT OF THE COMFORT RUT

The problem with continuing to always live within our comfort zone is that it effectively blocks us from any form of personal growth. The only way we can grow is to strike out and make changes. We can't do that if we're stuck in a rut of comfort.

Being afraid to venture outside our comfort zone seriously inhibits our quality of life. We must be willing to grow beyond the need for any particular comfort in order to achieve an even greater comfort. By giving up the satiety value of high-fat foods, for example, we can attain the far greater comfort of enjoying superb health and freedom from the threat of cardiovascular disease.

To make that leap of faith requires only a willingness to venture out beyond our comfort zone into areas of new growth where we have never ventured before.

Far from feeling deprived or restricted, dozens of people we met who had adopted a cholesterol-lowering lifestyle reported that it was never necessary to sacrifice the enjoyment of taste. They simply enjoyed new and exciting taste experiences from different foods.

Others told us that after beginning a brisk, half-hour daily walk, they became so addicted to the exhiliarating "high" they experienced afterwards, that they actively sought out other health-enhancing activities that made them feel even better. Instead of being addicted to their comfort zone, they became addicted to the even greater comfort of possessing high-level wellness.

All this adds up to a cogent argument against the almost

universal assumption that most Americans are unwilling or unable to adopt and stay with a cholesterol-lowering lifestyle.

WE'RE HARDIER THAN WE THINK

Most of us are far stronger and hardier and more flexible than we give ourselves credit for. Most of us have the potential to become survivors—for example, to survive being lost for days in the wilderness rather than to give up and die. Nor are we easily intimidated by mild inconveniences or by mental or physical exertion. Most of us are thoroughly capable of mobilizing the perseverence and commitment we need to survive. This means that we *can* choose to overcome the risk of heart disease rather than giving up and continuing to indulge in health risks that may speed our early demise.

Motivational studies have found that health advisories alone don't make people change. But people *are* powerfully motivated by concern for their health and the majority *are* willing to step outside their comfort zone.

Actually, one doesn't need to step very far outside the present comfort zone to adopt the Easy-Does-It Plan. For those willing to make a few additional changes, our Chol-Tamer Plan should provide swifter feedback. And for those committed to making fundamental rather than superficial changes, the Blockbuster Plan should provide the most positive benefits and the fastest cholesterol drop.

It's important to realize that each of these cholesterol-lowering plans is not merely a diet and exercise program but an entirely new philosophy of life and health. Each plan puts health high on our list of priorities. And the numerous health benefits we experience keep us permanently upbeat, positive and optimistic.

Motivational studies show that people who are winners make changes spontaneously. Professional counseling, or joining a support group, does not always have a significant impact on motivating people to change. Over 51 per cent of all changes are made by just doing it.

TO DO IT, YOU DO IT

That's all there is to making changes. To do it, you do it! And do it now! Don't put off starting until after Thanksgiving or Christmas. New Year's resolutions are seldom kept.

Nor should you allow lack of time to deter you. We all have too much to do and too little time to do it in. Which explains the popularity of popping a pill. Many doctors find it faster to write a prescription than to take the time to explain to patients how to lower their cholesterol by natural means.

Yet each of us has the same 24 hours in each day, and most of us find several hours each day to watch TV. If you're in this fix, consider buying an exercise bicycle and get your work-out while watching the tube. Create additional free time by cutting out all non-essential activity that is not inspiring or humorous, or that fails to benefit your health.

As you read on, you'll find tips to help you speed food preparation and still avoid using convenience and packaged foods. So unlike most other cholesterol books, this book is frankly designed to help cultivate your positive take-charge qualities. Step by step, each of the natural Cholesterol Cutter techniques that follow is designed to help tap into your personal resources so that you become a true winner at the cholesterol-lowering game.

SMOKING MUST GO

If you are among the 30 per cent of adult Americans who still smoke, you can prove you're a winner right now by becoming a non-smoker.

Smoking is a suicidal, health-wrecking habit that raises total and LDL cholesterol and suppresses HDL. According to the American Health Foundation, each two cigarettes smoked elevate total cholesterol one point for a period of 24 hours. Smoking is a major cause of artery injury, arterial plaque, high blood pressure, angina and coronary/artery spasm. It also constricts arteries in the legs causing claudication that can lead to gangrene and amputation. Smoking is also likely to increase risk of a blood clot that could directly trigger a fatal heart attack or stroke.

No one can really lower his cholesterol successfully until he has quit smoking for good. Moreover, there is no time to lose. The longer one has smoked, the greater the likelihood of serious blockage in the coronary arteries. Recent studies have also indicated that these same health risks can arise from passive smoking, that is inhaling the smoke from someone else's cigarettes.

Lack of space prevents us from giving a complete stop-smoking strategy. Yet a recent study by Dr. Michael C. Fiore of the University of Wisconsin found that smokers who quit cold turkey, and on their own, have a success rate almost twice that of those who enroll in an organized program.

Nevertheless, Dr. Fiore acknowledges that some really hard core smokers could benefit from smoking cessation programs. These include programs such as Smokenders and the non-commercial stop-smoking clinics sponsored by the American Cancer Society, American Lung Association, American Heart Association and the Seventh Day Adventists.

HAVE YOUR DOCTOR ORDER YOU TO STOP SMOKING

Some former smokers report that having their doctor issue a strongly-worded ultimatum to stop smoking immediately supplied all the impetus they needed to quit smoking on their own.

Additionally, many stop-smoking authorities advise switching from cigarettes to chewing a nicotine-based gum like Nicorettes. Also available are transdermal nicotine patches which deliver a low level of nicotine to aid in overcoming withdrawal symptoms without smoking.

For an easier withdrawal from the nicotine habit, cut back on caffeine (see CC # 15) at the same time that you cut back on smoking. Coffee actually exacerbates nicotine withdrawal symptoms like nervousness and insomnia. And don't rely on switching to low-tar or low-yield cigarettes. Surveys show that they merely increase the craving for more cigarettes.

Most people smoke because nicotine intensifies their alertness and arousal, and it creates a feeling of pleasure while subduing their level of pain and anxiety. Yet smokers fail to realize that regular daily exercise (see CC # 12), such as a brisk 45-minute walk, provides exactly the same level of arousal and alertness, and the same feeling of pleasure and freedom from pain and anxiety as smoking does. (All smokers should have their physician's approval before taking up exercise.)

Many other steps to help you quit smoking are available in books, or are taught in the clinics. However, you should not let fear of gaining weight deter you from ceasing to smoke. To equal the health risk of smoking, you'd have to be 120 pounds overweight. And any weight gain during this period is only temporary.

The benefits of ceasing to smoke start to appear within 24 hours. The natural abilities to taste and smell quickly return, coughing ceases, sleep improves, and virtually everyone feels incredible relief. Furthermore, in a recent study at the University of Florida, researchers found that in a group of women who stopped smoking, average HDL levels rose ten points in 30 days. But the best news is that two years after you cease to smoke, your risk of heart disease will have dropped to almost the same level as that of a lifetime non-smoker.

USE AVERSION THERAPY
TO GET BACK ON TRACK

What if, during a weak moment, you light up a cigarette again or eat a high-fat snack?

Whether it's smoking, food or exercise, if you do slip up, you can use aversion therapy immediately to get back on track.

To do that: Stop! Take six deep breaths! And begin all over again! One weak moment isn't going to stop you from following a lifetime of new health-building habits. One cigarette, or one hot dog, won't make that much difference. The important thing is not to take a second cigarette, nor to continue to indulge in high-risk foods.

We tend to become discouraged when we feel hungry, fatigued, lonely or tense. Most people go on an eating or a smoking binge in response to stress or negative moods. Whenever you feel this way, bolster your motivation by reading through this entire Cholesterol Cutter #1 section again. Then turn to CC # 16: Defuse Stress With Deep Muscle Relaxation.

Above all, avoid deliberate cheating. Cheating makes you feel guilty, an unnecessary negative emotion that undermines your winning spirit. If you find yourself in a social situation where you don't want to offend your hostess, you may occasionally fall off your diet. But compensate by cutting back on fat still more for the next few days. And do get back on track right away.

You can also use aversion therapy to break an addiction. Let's say you can't pass an ice cream parlor without going inside and ordering a banana split. Next time you feel this way, Stop! Take six deep breaths! And relax!

Then walk up to the ice cream parlor door—and turn right around and walk away again. Go about 30 yards. Stop! And take six deep breaths! Then repeat the entire routine. Repeat it ten times in all.

As this powerful technique builds fresh neural pathways in your mind, the old addiction will fade away.

CHAPTER SEVEN

The Dietary Approach— How to Eat Away Cholesterol

Like most American youngsters, Gregory Putnam grew up on a diet of colas, chips, ice cream, hot dogs, hamburgers, mayonnaise, cheese and white bread. As an adult, he continued to slather his meals with thick pats of butter and sour cream. A huge dollop of ice cream crowned every dessert. Each day, Gregory consumed the equivalent of one and-a-half sticks of butter in the form of fats and oils.

By his 38th birthday, Gregory was 35 pounds overweight and his wife was worried about his cholesterol level. After months of cajoling, Gregory visited his doctor and took a full Heart Disease Risk Profile blood test.

When the doctor read Gregory's test printout, he looked

concerned. Gregory's total cholesterol was a scary 270 mgs/ dl. His LDL was 190 mgs/dl., his HDL a bare 40, his VLDL was also 40, and his triglycerides a high 202. His total cholesterol/HDL ratio was a high-risk 6.75 while his blood pressure was moderately elevated at 145/92.

"Your risk factors show a strong probability of having a heart attack by your early fifties," the doctor warned. "That's if you don't get a stroke or cancer or diabetes first."

"But if you're willing to undo thirty years of incorrect eating," the doctor went on, "you can regain your health and probably live to be ninety. Food got you into this. And food is the one best way to turn your cholesterol levels around."

HEART-SMART EATING

Manipulating cholesterol levels by lowering the fat content of the diet, and by increasing fiber, is far safer than using drugs, the doctor told Gregory.

"A diet low in saturated fat and cholesterol is the safest and quickest way to lower these cholesterol levels," the doctor said." We all need small amounts of fat. But the quantities of fat that most Americans eat is a hazard to health."

The doctor explained that lowering fat in the diet while increasing fiber is the most powerful and direct way to lower cholesterol. Reducing the total amount of fat in the diet lowers total cholesterol along with LDL, VLDL and triglycerides levels. Cutting back on saturated fat will also send LDL plummetting in most people. And for those who prefer not to cut back too much on saturated fat, replacing saturated fat with monounsaturated fat also sends LDL reeling—in most people.

The doctor advised Gregory to cut his intake of total fat and saturated fat in half. At the same time, he was to double his intake of fiber.

Since most fat, and especially saturated fat, is derived from animal foods, and virtually all fiber is derived from plant foods, this translated into cutting his consumption of animal foods in half while doubling his intake of vegetables, fruits and whole grains.

AN EXCITING NEW WAY TO EAT

For Gregory, this was a whole new way of eating. He began to perceive dietary fat as sludge or grease that blocked the arteries in his heart and the capillary banks in his kidneys, and that suppressed his immune system which safeguarded him from infections and cancer.

Gregory's wife found that she could drastically reduce the amount of fat—by two-thirds in most recipes—without any reduction of eating pleasure. Gregory soon found that he enjoyed oatmeal and fresh fruits for breakfast far more than the fried eggs and bacon swimming in grease that he had eaten since childhood.

Lunch was often vegetable soup, with salad and a dressing based on plain, nonfat yogurt. His dinners focused on tasty entrees of vegetables, baked potatoes, and beans with rice, millet or barley. But now his meals weren't slathered in butter or cream.

After a few days, Gregory felt healthier than he had in years. In fact, he felt so good that it never occurred to him that he was restricted or deprived. Far from seeing his new eating plan as spartan or frugal, Gregory discovered a wealth of new gustatory pleasures in the honest taste of the fresh fruits, vegetables and grains that now made up most of his meals.

There were no limits on calories or quantity. Gregory's eating program allowed him three full meals a day with unlimited snacks in between. But instead of snacking on ice cream, chips, or cookies, he munched on plain popcorn, carrots, rice cakes, apples, bananas and other fruits.

THE AMAZING BENEFITS OF EATING CLEAN

After 60 days, Gregory felt like a new person. His relationship with his wife and children had improved and his boss had noticed his increased enthusiasm at work.

Gregory's weight had fallen by 20 pounds. And his cholesterol printout showed why. In 60 days, his total cholesterol had dropped 62 points to 208 mgs/dl. His LDL was down 54 points to only 136 mgs/dl., his HDL had actually risen two points to 42 mgs/dl., his VLDL had dropped 25 per cent to 30 mgs/dl., and his triglycerides had fallen 52 points to a much-improved 150 mgs/dl. Gregory's total cholesterol/HDL ratio, previously at 6.75, was now a much safer 4.9; and his blood pressure had fallen from 145/92 to a normal 130/87.

The eating program that Gregory's doctor had recommended was virtually identical to that of the 65-20-15 dietary formula of our Chol-Tamer Plan (65 per cent of calories from complex-carbohydrates; 20 from fat; and 15 from protein). From this point on, Gregory found that to keep his cholesterol dropping, he had to add exercise and some of the other Cholesterol Cutter techniques in this book.

True to form, Gregory's cholesterol levels proved to be dose-related. The more Cholesterol Cutter techniques he added to his program, the more his cholesterol levels improved. Each Cholesterol Cutter he added took his choles- terol down a few points more. Eventually, when his total cholesterol had stabilized at 170 mgs/dl., he switched to the 75-10-15 eating formula of our Blockbuster Plan. Within weeks, his total cholesterol had dropped to 150 mgs/dl.

While his holistic approach certainly paid off, it was Greg- ory's persistance in staying with the eating formulas that re- ally made the difference. Some people call it a "magic" formula. But it was that 65-20-15 eating program that alone took his total cholesterol down by 62 points in 60 days. And it was the 75-10-15 formula that helped carry it on down to a completely safe level.

DIETARY BLUEPRINT FOR LOW CHOLESTEROL

Eating more plant foods and fewer foods of animal origin, is what most of today's health advice is about. For several decades, cardiologists, nutritionists and health authorities— from the U.S. Surgeon Generals to the Senate Select Com- mittee on Nutrition and Human Needs, the National Re- search Council, the National Cancer Institute and at least 20 other top health advisory agencies in the U.S. and over- seas, have all endorsed a plant-based diet. Literally thousands of careful studies have implicated animal foods in the genesis of high cholesterol and chronic disease.

The still ongoing China Health Study reveals that a plant- based diet is completely safe and infinitely more healthful than one based on animal foods. The study's authors have concluded that there are multiple benefits from eating a plant-based diet and that 80-90 per cent of the ideal diet should consist of plant foods.

Until relatively recent times our ancestors had difficulty in obtaining enough dietary fat. The few animals they ate were lean and sinewy wild game. And like modern beans and grains, their wild vegetables were low in fats and oils.

Nowadays, the wild game of our ancestors has been replaced by feedlot-raised cattle pumped full of growth hormones and stuffed with corn. Corn-fed animals, it has been found, produce huge amounts of arachidonic acid, a fatty acid that, when consumed by humans, increases the tendency of platelets to form blood clots and to precipitate a heart attack or stroke. The flesh of feedlot animals is also high in palmitic fatty acid, a long-chain fatty acid known to be a promoter of high cholesterol.

NUTRITIONAL WISDOM FROM THE EXPERTS

In fact, a composite of the dietary advice dispensed by each of the nation's top health advisory agencies during recent years provides the following overall picture of the most healthful diet for humans.

- Americans should lose no time in cutting by half or more their daily intake of calories of fat and protein from animal sources; and they should at least double their daily consumption of fruits, vegetables and whole grains.
- Saturated fat has been found one-and-one-half to three times more capable of raising cholesterol levels and blocking arteries than dietary cholesterol itself. The principal sources of saturated fat are organ meats, all fatty meats and luncheon meats, animal fats of all kinds, lard and beef tallow, whole milk dairy products, cheese, butter and ice cream.
- Polyunsaturated oils, such as safflower and corn oils,

once thought to be a safe substitute for saturated fat, have now been found to lower HDL along with LDL; to be associated with artery injury through free radical activity; and also to be linked to immunosuppression. Today, monounsaturated fats like olive and canola oils, are considered safer to eat.

• The same high-fat diet that causes high cholesterol, heart disease and stroke has also been directly linked to hypertension, diabetes, cancer of the breast, colon, prostate and liver, renal disease, obesity and blood clots. Many authorities today consider the AHA's top limit of 30 per cent of calories from fat to be far too high and they recommend a fat intake of only 10-20 per cent of calories.

From the National Institutes of Health to the National Academy of Sciences, the advice is loud and clear: we should replace much of our excessively high intake of animal fat and protein with coarse plant foods. We should eat twice as many vegetables as fruits and include plenty of beans, dark-green and yellow-orange vegetables, cruciferous family vegetables (broccoli, brussels sprouts, cauliflower etc.,) and green peppers, onions and garlic.

Not a word ever appears about increasing your intake of eggs, meat, poultry, fish or dairy products—merely some suggestions that fish, poultry or nonfat dairy products may be safer substitutes for meat. (Because it contains blood-thinning Omega-3 fats, fish is probably the least harmful of all flesh foods. But fish is still high in animal protein, may contain saturated fat and cholesterol, and has zero fiber.)

ENDING CONFUSION ABOUT WHAT TO EAT

In scientific terms, the advice is obviously sound and unmistakable. But in practice, how do we measure out 20 per cent of calories on our plate?

Befuddling the whole issue is that every food consists of carbohydrates, fats and protein, and every fat is composed of saturated, polyunsaturated and monounsaturated fats. What we call a carbohydrate is simply a food that consists predominently of carbohydrates but that also contains some fat and some protein. A protein food consists predominently of amino acids (the building blocks of protein) together with some fat and carbohydrates. And a saturated fat is a lipid that contains more saturated fat than polyunsaturated or monounsaturated fats—yet all three are represented.

Knowing more about each of these three food components is a big help in learning how to use them to fight cholesterol. All foods break down into their carbohydrate, protein and fat components.

Carbohydrates

Complex carbohydrates refers to any plant food still in the same whole, unfragmented, unprocessed and unrefined state in which it grew in nature. In this unchanged, natural condition, the still-living cells are enclosed in a membrane of cellulose. Most complex carbohydrates, such as beans, seeds, vegetables, fruits or grains, will grow if planted in the ground. Hence they are also known as "living foods." Also classified as complex carbohydrates are mildly-processed grains like whole wheat flour and oatmeal which retain many of the qualities of live foods during their relatively short shelf life.

Complex Carbohydrates Are Cholesterol Fighters

Complex carbohydrates are the only foods to contain any appreciable fiber. This vital cholesterol-fighter is almost non-existant in fats, animal protein and refined carbohydrates

Simple or refined carbohydrates are produced when complex carbohydrates like grain, sugar or rice is milled and stripped of its germ and cellulose walls, and is transformed into white flour, white sugar or white rice. In this way, carbohydrates are refined to increase their shelf life for greater profit to the food industry. (No one seems to care that eating them may help to shorten your life.)

The refining process destroys almost all fiber together with most B vitamins, magnesium, zinc, manganese and other nutrients essential to the health of heart and arteries. Only empty calories remain.

Since they lack cell walls, refined carbohydrates are absorbed rapidly by the digestive system, sending a burst of sugar into the blood stream that sets blood sugar and insulin levels soaring. The effect on the liver is similar to that of diabetes. *The net result is to elevate both cholesterol and triglycerides levels.*

Obviously, we should stay as far away as possible from all refined carbohydrates. We must never forget that all types of sweeteners are also refined carbohydrates including honey, molasses, brown or white sugar, extracted fructose and beet sugar, dextrose, malt, galactose, sorghum, sorbitol and xylose. Dried fruits, though high in fiber, are very concentrated in fruit sugar and should be eaten only in small quantities.

The body's need for refined carbohydrates is absolute zero. Yet manufacturers persist in including them in virtually every type of prepared, processed, manufactured and canned food.

Refined carbohydrates exist in almost every processed food and in most commercial cakes, pies and baked goods. Most commercial "whole wheat" breads actually contain mostly white flour as well as too much sugar, fats and oils. Even alcohol is a refined carbohydrate. And while white rice isn't quite as bad as other refined carbohydrates, always choose whole grain or brown rice when you can.

Eat the Right Carbohydrates

The carbohydrates that fight cholesterol are complex carbohydrates. Due to their high fiber content, they are not exceptionally high in calories. A medium sized potato has only 100 calories (but 300 calories if we plaster it with sour cream and 500 calories if we fry it). It is what we *put on* complex carbohydrates that makes some plant foods seem high in calories. As a result, millions of people still erroneously believe that corn tortillas, spaghetti or plain baked potatoes are fattening and that cereals, bread and pasta are high in calories.

Although it may take several hours to digest and release their calories, complex carbohydrates are still the ideal high-energy foods.

How many complex carbohydrates should one eat when following the Chol-Tamer Plan, for example? The answer is simple. Provided you stay within the permitted amounts of animal-derived foods and other fats and oils, the rest of your diet can consist entirely of complex carbohydrates. Since there is no calorie limit, you can eat all the complex carbohydrates you like—virtually unlimited amounts of fruits, vegetables, whole grains and legumes. The only caution is to eat twice as many vegetables as fruits, and to include plenty of grains and legumes.

Protein

Protein consists of 22 amino acids which, in various combinations, form the building blocks of all our cells. They are also essential to almost every human function. Since our bodies can synthesize only 13 amino acids from food, the remaining nine—known as essential amino acids (EAAs)—must be obtained directly from the diet. Almost all animal-derived foods supply all nine EAAs. But no single plant food contains whole protein. Nonetheless, protein needs can easily be met on a plant-based diet by including a variety of vegetables, beans and whole grains each day. Those amino acids lacking in one plant food are supplied by another.

Complementing almost any whole grain with a legume results in whole protein. For example, a combination of corn and beans or rice and beans or whole grain bread with pure peanut butter (without added fat or sugar) results in protein equal in quality to any obtainable from meat, eggs or dairy products. Nor is it considered necessary to eat the grains and legumes at the same meal. Provided you eat a variety of vegetables, legumes and grains during the day, you should have ample amounts of complete protein. Furthermore, grains and beans are much cheaper sources of protein than meat.

The American Obsession with Protein

Since the 1950s, Americans have been obsessed with the myth that only eggs, meat and dairy products provide high quality protein and that we would all become sick if we didn't eat an abundance of animal foods. In most households and restaurants, meat and chicken still dominate every dinner plate with a few token vegetables or some rice placed on the side.

113

Not surprisingly, we are in the midst of a national epidemic of high cholesterol and heart disease, stroke, cancer, broken hips and renal disease. One problem has always been that animal protein is usually found only in close association with large amounts of saturated fat and cholesterol. It is often difficult to eat meat or whole milk dairy products for their protein content alone without also consuming excessive amounts of saturated fat and cholesterol.

But in recent years, increasing evidence has emerged to show that, even when separated entirely from fat and cholesterol, animal protein alone has been linked to a significant increase in human cholesterol levels. Preliminary findings from the China Health Study and others appear to indicate that animal protein by itself increases total cholesterol quite apart from any association with saturated fat or cholesterol.

Over the years, evidence from an increasing number of nutritional and epidemiological studies has also shown strong links between a high intake of animal protein and incidence of heart disease, stroke, kidney disease, osteoporosis, and cancer of the breast, prostate, rectum, pancreas, kidney, liver and endometrium. Additionally, numerous animal studies have confirmed that when lab animals are fed twice as much protein as required for normal growth, incidence of all these cancers and other diseases increases significantly. A growing body of evidence is also emerging to show that animal protein promotes growth in tumors of all types.

Plant Protein Is Healthier

Human studies are also showing that it is the *source* of the protein that counts. All the damage appears to emanate from animal protein. Partly that's because it is easy to overdose on protein from animal sources. U.S. government statistics show that both the average American male, and the average youngster, consume almost twice the RDA for protein.

Compared to the RDA of eight to nine per cent of calories from protein, most Americans eat 15 per cent, which is close to the upper limit that the body can tolerate. Put another way, while the UNICEF RDA for protein is eight-tenths of a gram per kilo of body weight (which averages out to 55 grams for the average man, and 46 grams for the average woman), the average American consumes 90 grams of protein per day of which 70 per cent is from animal sources.

When these excessive amounts of protein break down in the body, they create huge amounts of nitrogen by-products such as urea and ammonia. This process draws down the body's reserves of magnesium and calcium. Not only are these minerals essential to heart health but the resulting deficiency is also largely responsible for much of the osteoporosis, or bone loss, suffered each year by millions of older American women.

No such ill effects have ever been observed from eating vegetable protein. All vegetables, grains and legumes contain adequate amounts of the EAAs to meet nutritional requirements. In fact, the protein content of many beans is higher than that of comparable amounts of meat.

Plant foods particularly high in protein include lentils, garbanzo, kidney and soy beans, tofu, sunflower seeds, wheat germ, brown rice, millet, barley and oatmeal. Plant proteins are simply complex carbohydrates with an above-average protein content. Since all complex carbohydrates are also high in fiber, when we obtain our protein from complex carbohydrates, we also enjoy the cholesterol-lowering benefits of the fiber they contain. Carbohydrates are also far superior to any animal protein as an energy source.

The conclusion is that we should obtain as much protein as we can from complex carbohydrates and we should minimize our dependance on animal foods for our protein requirements.

Protein Guidelines for the Three Cholesterol-Lowering Plans

Each of our three cholesterol-lowering programs provides an ample supply of protein.

The Easy-Does-It Plan, with its 55-30-15 formula, permits up to six ounces of very lean meat, fish or skinless poultry per day of which not more than three ounces may consist of meat. Alternatively, proportionate amounts of plain, nonfat yogurt, skim milk or egg whites could be substituted for some of the flesh foods. This is certainly a generous amount when you consider that six ounces of chicken supplies 120 per cent of the RDA for protein while six ounces of flounder provides 77 per cent. The remainder is derived from plant sources such as grains and beans.

The Chol-Tamer Plan, with its 65-20-15 formula, limits animal-derived foods to three-and-one-half ounces of fish or skinless poultry daily. Alternatively, proportionate amounts of plain, nonfat yogurt, skim milk or egg whites may be substituted for some of the flesh foods. Three-and-a-half ounces of chicken supplies 70 per cent of the RDA for protein while the same amount of flounder supplies 41 per cent. The remainder is easily met from plant sources.

Recognizing that animal protein alone can raise cholesterol, the Blockbuster Plan, with its 75-10-15 formula, obtains the majority of its protein requirements from plant sources. Animal protein is limited to one eight-ounce cup of plain, nonfat yogurt or skim milk daily or, if preferred, up to three egg whites instead. All other protein needs are met from plant sources. Since the average 2,000 calorie diet of mixed vegetables, grains and legumes supplies 50-70 grams of protein per day, this easily exceeds the RDA for protein. The single cup of yogurt alone supplies 30 per cent of the RDA for protein. The only caution is to be sure to consume most of your calories in the form of whole grains, legumes and vegetables each day.

All protein requirements discussed here apply only to healthy adults. Diabetics and others may have special requirements. Pregnant and nursing women also generally require additional protein while infants and young children may also require additional fat.

While the protein allowances of each of our cholesterol-lowering plans may seem high, we must remember that in the Chol-Tamer and Blockbuster Plans, the majority is derived from harm-free plant sources.

Fat

Reducing our total fat intake is central to any effort to lower cholesterol. This is hardly surprising when you consider that the average American eats 66 pounds of fats and oils per year and derives approximately 40 per cent of calories from fat. Half of those fat calories are from saturated fat, the most potent promoter of cholesterol in existence. Every year, the average American eats 11 gallons of ice cream, 79 pounds of beef, 261 eggs, and consumes the equivalent of one stick of butter in the form of fats and oils each day. Many eat much more.

Any diet from which 35-40 per cent or more of calories are derived from fat is classified as a *high-fat diet*. A *moderate-fat diet* derives 20 percent or less of calories from fat; and a *low-fat diet* derives ten per cent, or less, of calories from fat.

Many of the world's top nutritionists and cardiologists are suggesting that fat intake be cut to a maximum of 25 per cent of calories, or to 15 per cent for people with dangerously high cholesterol. The NAS has recommended cutting saturated fat consumption in half. And a report in the *Journal of the American Medical Association* (March 23, 1990) stated that we could stop cholesterol deposits from building up in the arteries by keeping total fat intake to 25 per cent of calories or less.

Meanwhile, the universal advice of more advanced nutritionists, and the preventive medicine school, is to limit fat intake to a maximum of 20 per cent of calories (a moderate-fat diet) or to ten per cent or less (a low-fat diet).

Hold the Fat

To lower cholesterol, it is as important to lower *total* fat intake as it is to lower intake of saturated or other types of fat. Hence we should be wary about advice to replace saturated fat with polyunsaturated fat; or to replace polyunsaturated fat with mono-unsaturated fat. All fat has nine calories per gram. And while some fats are certainly more dangerous than others, replacing one fat with another does nothing to lower total fat consumption.

We suggest being skeptical of advice to eat more fats or oils for any reason whatsoever. That includes consuming additional oil to prevent dry skin. The answer here is to use a topical cream or moisturizer and to drink lots of water.

Using fish as a substitute for meat, eggs or whole milk dairy foods is generally good advice, but eating beans and rice instead would probably lower cholesterol more. Nor should you pour additional olive oil on your salad in the belief that it will lower cholesterol. While olive oil is a good substitute for regular mayonnaise, or a dressing high in poly-unsaturated fats, it is still 100 per cent pure fat. A liberal application of olive oil can boost the total fat content of a salad from around five per cent of calories to over 60 per cent.

Fat Allotments for the Three Cholesterol Lowering Plans

Nutritionists measure the fat content of food in one of two ways: 1) as a percentage of total calories; or 2) in grams.

Fat is expressed as a percentage of calories because the actual amount of fat we consume depends on the number of calories we eat. On a diet in which 30 per cent of calories is derived from fat, a woman eating 1,600 calories daily would take in 53 grams of fat while a man eating 2,400 calories would get 80 grams of fat.

The following table shows the maximum number of grams of fat a person would consume while following the Easy-Does-It Plan (up to 30 per cent of calories from fat); the

Total Calories in Diet	Grams of Fat Consumed		
	Easy-Does-It 30%	Chol-Tamer 20%	Blockbuster 10%
1200	40	26	13
1400	47	31	16
1600	53	35	18
1800	60	40	20
2000	67	45	23
2200	73	49	25
2400	80	54	27
2600	86	58	29
2800	94	62	31
3000	100	66	33

Chol-Tamer Plan (up to 20 per cent of calories from fat); and the Blockbuster Plan (up to ten per cent of calories from fat).

Remember that just one tablespoon of olive oil, butter or mayonnaise contains 14 grams of fat and one ounce of fat is approximately 29 grams.

How to Calculate the Fat Content of Any Processed Food

How can you calculate the percentage of calories from fat for any food? Most processed foods nowadays carry a label listing the number of grams of fat, and the total calories per serving. From these two factors, the following simple formula gives you the percentage of calories from fat.

$$\frac{\text{grams of fat} \times 9}{\text{total calories}} \times 100 = \text{percentage of calories from fat}$$

Example: a jar of natural peanut butter has a fat content of 9 grams and a calorie content of 200 per serving.

$$\frac{9 \times 9}{200} \times 100 = 40.5$$

The simple calculation ($9 \times 9 = 81$ divided by 200 = .405 $\times$ 100 = 40.5) shows that this peanut butter derives 40.5 per cent of its calories from fat.

Another example: a can of chicken soup has two grams of fat and 60 calories per serving.

$$\frac{2 \times 9}{60} \times 100 = 30$$

This soup, which contains some eggs and margarine, derives 30 per cent of its calories from fat.

Applying this formula reveals some surprising facts about the heart-healthiness of foods. For example, although whole milk is only four per cent fat by weight, it turns out that 48 per cent of its calories come from fat. Two per cent milk gets about 38 per cent of calories from fat while one per cent milk still derives some 18 per cent of calories from fat. By comparison, turkey breast gets about 5 per cent of calories from fat.

Knowing the percentage of calories from fat allows you to compare the total fat content of any one food with that of another food or brand. Nowadays, it's not unusual to see fat-conscious shoppers busily punching grams and calories onto pocket calculators as they seek to find food with the lowest fat content.

By doing the same, you can easily compare the fat content of most types of processed supermarket foods.

Cutting Just Two Tablespoons of Fat Per Day May Lower Your Cholesterol

For the average man to cut fat intake from 40 per cent of calories to 30 per cent requires cutting out 28 grams of fat per day (approximately equal to one ounce or two table-spoons). To drop to 20 per cent requires eliminating twice as much dietary fat. Knowing how many tablespoons of fat must go helps in visualizing your goal. But only bottled oils or sticks of butter can be doled out in tablespoons. Most other fats are mixed up with protein and carbohydrate and are often invisible.

To help assess which fats, and how much of each, to get rid of, here are the pros and cons of each of the five principal fat types in the American diet.

Incidentally, you needn't be afraid of cutting too much fat out of your diet. The only essential fatty acids that the body cannot synthesize are linoleic and linolenic acids. Our nutritional needs for these fatty acids can easily be supplied by one-to-two teaspoons of poly-unsaturated fat per day. This amount is easily met by almost any low-fat diet that includes grains and beans.

Saturated Fat—A Villain of Formidable Proportions

Saturated fat consists of molecules with a carbon skeleton filled or saturated with the maximum possible number of hydrogen atoms. This makes saturated fats solid at room temperature, and they remain solidified in the human body. Because they provoke the liver to manufacture one-and-one-half to three times their weight in cholesterol, saturated fats are the single most powerful elevator of total cholesterol.

High levels of saturated fat, cholesterol and animal protein frequently occur together, particularly in meat, cheese and butter. However, some pressed vegetable oils contain high levels of saturated fat. For example, 92 per cent of coconut oil is saturated fat, as is 86 per cent of palm kernel oil, 51 per cent of palm oil, and 27 per cent of cottonseed oil.

Among animal foods with the highest saturated fat levels are: organ meats (liver, brains, kidneys, giblets, sweetbreads, etc.); red meats (especially beef, pork and lamb); whole milk dairy products (butter, cheese, ice cream, sour cream and milk); bacon, sausage and processed luncheon meats; and any foods made with, or cooked in, beef tallow, lard or tropical oils. Coconut also contains appreciable amounts of saturated fat.

Fortunately, tropical oils are being withdrawn from many U.S., foods. Yet the standard American diet remains dangerously high in saturated fat, with up to 20 per cent of calories derived from saturated fat alone.

In our three cholesterol-lowering plans, saturated fat is cut to a maximum of ten per cent of calories in the Easy-Does-

It Plan; to a maximum of seven per cent in the Chol-Tamer Plan; and to a maximum of two-and-a-half per cent in the Blockbuster Plan. While one can only estimate these amounts, these targets are easily met by avoiding all or most of the foods just mentioned. All skin should be removed from poultry and any visible fat should be cut from meat.

Polyunsaturated Fats—A Dietary Trade-Off

Polyunsaturated fats have a carbon skeleton in which 4 or more spots remain unsaturated by hydrogen atoms. This makes them liquid at room temperature. The majority are omega-6 oils of vegetable origin which occur naturally in grains, seeds, nuts and legumes. The largest source of polyunsaturated fats are pressed vegetable oils made from grains, legumes and seeds.

Among the most common are corn, safflower, soybean, cottonseed and sesame seed oils. These oils are widely used in frying and in baked goods, and are a common ingredient in prepared foods of every kind.

For many years, Americans were urged to replace saturated fats with polyunsaturated vegetable oils. The rationale was that polyunsaturated oils lowered total cholesterol. More recent research has shown that this effect is achieved by the fatty acid oleate which lowers both LDL and HDL together. Since lowering HDL is undesirable, the popularity of polyunsaturated fats has declined. Today, most health advisory agencies recommend monounsaturated oils as a healthier substitute for saturated fats.

When used in cooking, the high temperatures cause the double bonds of polyunsaturated oils to combine with oxygen to form peroxides. Oxidization can also occur more slowly at room temperature. The result is that exposure to air or heat can render polyunsaturated fats chemically rancid. These oxidized lipids then release free radicals in the form of molecules containing unpaired electrons. In the blood stream, they become highly reactive agents capable of injuring cells in artery walls or of changing the DNA in body cells to promote cancer.

Since every plant cell contains a variety of antioxidants such as Vitamins C and E, selenium and carotenoids, all of which nullify free radical activity, there is no danger from free radicals when eating fresh fruits, vegetables, grains, legumes or other plant foods. The body also contains a system of enzyme antioxidants which are perfectly capable of destroying any free radicals introduced into the body in natural foods, and even of repairing any damage they cause.

Polyunsaturated Oils May Compromise Health

The problem arises when man tampers with plant foods and squeezes them under pressure to extract their oils. Unlike the plants from which they derive, vegetable oils are 100 per cent fat. Consuming these oils in the diet can cause obesity as easily as a well-marbled steak.

Recent studies at the University of Alabama have strongly suggested that foods fried in polyunsaturated oils can injure artery walls. Numerous animal experiments have also suggested that consuming more than ten per cent of calories from polyunsaturated fats can increase cancer risk, suppress immunity and increase risk of gallstones.

Researchers have also concluded that no population that consumes a high level of polyunsaturated fats has a good health record. In fact, no human population has ever lived on a polyunsaturated fat-rich diet. This has caused most nutritionists to suggest limiting polyunsaturated fat intake to a maximum of ten per cent of dietary calories.

Most health advisory agencies are also wary of any advice to replace saturated fat with polyunsaturated oils. Rather, they suggest limiting intake of polyunsaturated oils as you limit intake of total fat. If you *must* sauté foods, use monounsaturated oils like olive and canola instead. They remain stable when exposed to light or heat.

Polyunsaturated oils are limited to a maximum of ten per cent of calories in our Easy-Does-It Plan; to seven per cent in the Chol-Tamer Plan; and to three per cent in the Blockbuster Plan. Since all of the body's needs for polyunsaturated fats are easily met by grains and legumes in the diet, this suggests that these pressed vegetable oils should be used very, *very* sparingly, if at all.

Monounsaturated Fats—And the Mediterranean Connection

Monounsaturated fats have a carbon skeleton with room for more hydrogen atoms only at one location. Monounsaturated oils are pressed from olives, rapeseed, peanuts and avocadoes to form olive oil, canola or rapeseed oil, peanut oil and avocado oil.

The benefits of monounsaturated fats were first revealed by the Seven Countries Study, a landmark epidemiological study that monitored 16 groups of healthy men in seven countries ranging from Japan to the U.S., east Finland, Spain and the Greek island of Crete. In all seven countries it was found that the higher the saturated fat intake, the higher the cholesterol level and the greater the death rate from heart disease. But while the heart attack rate was 628 per 10,000 among the Finns, 424 per 10,000 among Americans, and from 50-to-317 per 10,000 among four other nationalities, the rate in Crete was zero. Out of 655 men actually monitored in Crete, not one died of heart disease.

Investigations showed that although the Cretans ate as much fat as men in other countries, virtually their entire consumption consisted of olive oil. Other Mediterranean countries in which this mono-unsaturated oil was widely used, also showed lower rates of heart disease. Researchers soon found out that olive oil lowers total cholesterol by reducing LDL without lowering HDL.

Oils That Are Friendly to Arteries

More recent studies by Scott Grundy, Ph.D., at the University of Texas Southwest Medical Center, Dallas, have shown that monounsaturated fats can lower both total and LDL cholesterol while, at the same time, maintaining the HDL level, or even raising it slightly. Other studies have revealed that monounsaturated oils lower LDL more effectively than polyunsaturated oils without suppressing the HDL level. Thus far, neither olive nor canola oils have shown any tendency to produce free radical damage, to injure artery walls, to cause cancer or to suppress immunity.

Since some animal studies have suggested that peanut oil is less safe than olive or canola oil, these two are generally recommended as replacements for saturated or polyunsaturated fats. Despite these seeming advantages, however, all mono-unsaturated oils are still 100 per cent pure fat and over-consumption can easily lead to overweight.

Either olive or canola oil can be used to replace saturated or poly-unsaturated fats in most recipes. Canola oil has the advantage of being tasteless, and is thus preferable for baked goods.

Our Easy-Does-It Plan allows up to ten per cent of calories

from monounsaturated oils, with a limit of approximately seven per cent for the Chol-Tamer Plan, and four-and-a-half per cent for the Blockbuster Plan.

Partially-Hydrogenated Vegetable Oils—A Fat to Avoid

Partially-hydrogenated vegetable oils are manufactured under heat and pressure by saturating the double bonds in poly-unsaturated oils with more hydrogen. This alters the molecular structure of some of the oil's monounsaturated fat content from its naturally-occuring *cis* structure into a trans-fatty acid. Put another way, it transforms liquid oil into tub margarine.

As tropical oils were phased out in recent years, partially-hydrogenated vegetable oils were used instead in hundreds of processed foods from supermarket breads to cakes, cookies, crackers, baked goods, candy, egg substitutes, non-dairy creamers and in a wide variety of fried foods. They are most commonly found in margarine and shortening.

The body has absolutely zero need for partially-hydrogenated vegetable oils, and the sole reason for their existence is to increase food industry profits by making oils more solid and stable, by giving them a creamy texture, and by increasing their shelf life. The more solid and hydrogenated an oil is, the more trans-fatty acids it contains.

How safe, then, are these oils that do not exist in nature, and that give a poly-unsaturated fat more of the characteristics of saturated fat? More and more studies are suggesting that partially-hydrogenated oils are another man-made food product which can damage the body in one way or another. For one thing, the unnatural fatty acid isomers produced in the manufacturing process appear to inhibit the HDL's task of clearing cholesterol out of the arteries. Animal research has also shown a link between hydrogenated fats and tumor growth.

Researchers at the University of Wisconsin have suggested that the trans-fatty acids in partially-hydrogenated oils may block enzymes that control cholesterol metabolism. The effect is to inhibit secretion of cholesterol by the body resulting in an increase in total cholesterol.

In another recent study by Ronald Mensink and Martijn Katan at the Agricultural University of the Netherlands, 59 young men and women were each fed for three weeks a diet containing: 1) a trans-fatty acid; 2) a monounsaturated oil in a naturally-occurring *cis* form and; 3) a saturated fat. While those consuming the saturated fat showed the highest cholesterol levels, those eating the trans-fatty acid diet showed an increase in both total and LDL cholesterol that was markedly higher than in those eating the *cis* form of oil. The authors concluded that eating a trans-fatty acid was almost as unfavorable as eating saturated fat.

The purpose of this section is to suggest that margarine and all other foods containing partially-hydrogenated oils are best avoided.

• Fish Oils—Fats That Can Upgrade Your Nutrition

Omega-3 polyunsaturated oils found in fish and some seafoods are often touted as heart-healthy foods. This needs clarifying by stating that any health benefits appear to arise from *eating fish or seafood* itself and not necessarily from taking fish oil supplements in capsule form. Certain fish oils in liquid form, including cod liver oil, may be more likely to raise cholesterol than lower it. Hence fish itself is preferable.

Although fish and seafood contain saturated fat and cholesterol, population studies of fish-eating peoples such as Eskimos, Japanese, Icelanders and Norwegians, all show a below-average rate of heart disease. However, the benefits appear to emanate from the anti-coagulating properties of the fish oils rather than from any ability to lower cholesterol. By reducing the stickiness of blood platelets, these oils do lower the risk of heart disease. But they may also increase the risk of a hemorrhagic stroke.

From five-to-40 per cent of fat in fish and seafood consists of omega-3 fatty acids in the form of either eicosapentaenoic acid (EPA) or decosahexaenoic acid (DHA). These oils are most plentiful in cold water fish and seafood such as salmon, sardines, mackerel, whitefish, herring, white tuna, halibut, pompano and rainbow trout. Fish caught in deep oceans are probably best since those taken close to shore, in rivers or in lakes, may be contaminated with toxic wastes.

Some studies have shown that omega-3 oils may help to lower the liver's production of triglycerides and to reduce risk of several cancers. It is true that fish and seafood may contain less saturated fat than beef, pork or lamb. Yet they still do contain some of these lipids and they are still high in calories and in animal protein. Oily fish can also be fattening.

Their principal advantage is that they are a leaner substitute for beef or whole milk dairy foods. And their best use is as a replacement for red meat, eggs or poultry.

This makes fish and certain seafoods possibly the least harmful of all flesh foods. But you can still lower your cholesterol more by replacing fish with grains or beans than by replacing meat and poultry with fish. And proof is still lacking that eating more fish lowers cholesterol.

(Strict vegetarians and those who wish to avoid fish can still get ample amounts of omega-3 fats through the following excellent vegetable sources: ground flaxseed or flaxseed oil, canola oil, soy oil, purslane and spinach.)

Now that you've learned the principles of cholesterol nutrition, the following Cholesterol Cutter techniques will help you put them into action.

CHOLESTEROL CUTTER # 2:

OUTLAW THESE GREMLIN FOODS FROM YOUR DIET

Listed below are just about all the most common foods that, directly or indirectly, send cholesterol levels soaring. Some people may ask with dismay what is left to eat? All the foods they love are on this list.

Hence, to show this list to some people is to lose them entirely. But before getting discouraged, ask yourself what this list is *really* about. All the foods that this list suggests cutting back on have one thing in common. *They are virtually all rich, high-fat foods that form the core of the affluent Western diet*. We may believe we eat them to enjoy their taste. But motivational psychology has discovered that many people find emotional comfort in sweet or fatty foods while others choose them to enhance their social status.

Most Americans view beans and rice or vegetables as peasant food, as food that somehow doesn't measure up to what is considered socially acceptable in our affluent culture. All too often, plant-based foods are seen as fit only for people in Third World countries or for those who can't afford anything better.

We also eat these rich foods to conform to, and to share, what our friends and relatives eat and enjoy. Yet if we really analyzed it, very few meats, fish, poultry or seafood have any real, inherent taste. They have to be fried, broiled, grilled, charred, blackened, smoked or pickled first. Or we have to fill a bird with stuffing, or deep-fry it, or pour on sauces, gravy, butter or cream to impart any meaningful taste to most animal foods.

In re-evaluating our approach to food, the mental act of changing the way we look at food is a far greater stumbling block for most people than any actual addiction to taste. Changing our eating patterns is not so much a matter of switching to different foods as it is of explaining to all our family members and friends why we are suddenly eating foods that are different from theirs.

Seen from this perspective, cutting back on, or eliminating some of the foods in this section can usually be achieved smoothly and painlessly without straying very far from our comfort zone. Making it all easier is the realization that not a single food on this list contributes anything to our health. Some of the foods are downright hazardous. By cutting back on these foods, or by eliminating them altogether, we can take a giant step towards better health.

Here, then, is a frank and objective list of those foods which science has validated as being most responsible for raising cholesterol.

The Top Artery-Clogging Foods

• *Cholesterol-Booster #1: Organ Meats and Tropical Oils.*

All organ meats, whether from animal, fish or poultry— and especially brains, kidneys, giblets, liver, sweetbreads, gizzards or fish roe—rank among the most dangerous of foods. Four ounces of beef brains contain a frightening 1,900 mgs of cholesterol while four ounces of beef liver has 545 mgs of cholesterol and three grams of saturated fat.

Tropical oils such as palm oil, palm kernel oil, and coconut oil or cocoa butter are also excessively high in saturated fats. Although withdrawn from most U.S. foods, they may still be encountered.

• Cholesterol Booster #2: Red Meat

Many cuts of beef, pork, lamb and veal are two-thirds fat and one-third animal protein. Half of beef's fat consists of palmitic fatty acid, a powerful promoter of cholesterol. Even with the fat trimmed off, a four-ounce serving of red meat typically contains 100 mgs of cholesterol and a whopping 4.5 grams of saturated fat.

Meat industry spokesmen claim that today's beef is 27 per cent leaner, and pork 31 per cent leaner, than in 1976 when most meats were tested by the USDA. Even so, recent tests showed that a chuck roast of beef still had 2.8 grams of saturated fat per serving, compared to 3.8 in 1976, while the cholesterol content remained at the same 101 mgs. A piece of fairly lean meat today still has 28 times as much saturated fat as cholesterol.

Steak, hamburgers or lard (pork fat) are all excessively high in saturated fat while animal protein and red meat has been associated with risk of several types of cancer and with osteoporosis and renal disease.

• Cholesterol Booster #3: Whole Milk Dairy Products

Whole milk derives 45-50 per cent of calories from fat and a single cup contains 33 mgs of cholesterol and five grams of fat. Virtually all whole milk products are excessively high in saturated fat and cholesterol. Except for Vitamin A, butter contains little of any nutritional value yet derives nearly 100 per cent of calories from fat and two-thirds of that is saturated. A single tablespoon contains 36 mgs of cholesterol and 8.7 grams of saturated fat.

Low-fat dairy foods all contain some cholesterol while up to 40 per cent of their calories may come from fat. For example, two per cent milk doesn't mean two per cent of calories comes from fat. One-tenth of two per cent milk consists of milk solids and the rest is water. Take away the water and what you have left is 20 per cent fat by weight. This translates into 35-40 per cent of calories from fat. Even one per cent milk derives 18 per cent of calories from fat.

Yet regular cheese easily wins as the fattiest of dairy foods. Cheddar cheese gets 71 per cent of calories from fat, Swiss cheese 73 per cent, and Parmesan 58. Almost all hard cheeses are high in fat, including both regular mozzarella and ricotta. In fact, the harder the cheese, the higher the fat. Cheeseburgers and pizza are just as fat-laden.

Even "light," "slender," and "part-skim" cheeses are all high in cholesterol and the majority still derive a surprisingly high 45-56 per cent of calories from fat. Most cream cheese, which can be up to 90 per cent fat, should also be avoided.

• Cholesterol Booster #4: Cured and Processed Meats.

Salami, pepperoni and bologna are among the fattiest of luncheon meats with up to 80 per cent of calories derived from fat. All types of cured meats, from bacon to smoked ham, sausage, cold cuts, franks and hot dogs, are likely to send LDL levels soaring. Even "lite" deli foods like roast beef or lean baked ham often get 35 per cent of calories from fat. "Extra lean ham," with 29-32 per cent of calories from fat, may not be much better, and even turkey ham (using thighs) gets about one-fourth of its calories from fat.

Processed fish and poultry items are often high in saturated

133

fat. For instance, breaded chicken patties may contain skin, are often deep fried, and may get as much as half their calories from fat. Roughly half the fat in a chicken is in the skin and any type of ground chicken or turkey may contain skin. Likewise, breaded fish fillets are also usually deep-fried and may get half their calories from fat. For clean arteries, avoid any type of chicken fat or any food that includes chicken skin. You should also avoid duck or goose in any form.

• Cholesterol Booster #5: Eggs

According to egg industry sources, one large egg today contains 213 mgs of cholesterol rather than the 274 mgs shown in 1976 tests. Even so, two eggs still exceeds the AHA's daily cholesterol limit by 126 mgs. While not high in saturated fat, one egg still has 1.7 grams. And if your eggs are fried, fat intake skyrockets.

One problem is that, although invisible, eggs are extensively used in recipes, and in processed foods and baked goods. Anyone who is really serious about lowering cholesterol would do well to avoid all egg yolks, and any food containing them.

• Cholesterol Booster #6: Ice Cream

A half cup of ice cream contains 24 grams of fat, much of it saturated. Next time you're eyeing a hot fudge sundae, consider substituting nonfat frozen yogurt instead. Or try an ice popsicle or a frozen banana.

• Cholesterol Booster #7: Baked Goods, Candy and Chocolate

Huge amounts of saturated fat, and partially-hydrogenated vegetable oils, may be hidden in commercially-made pie crusts and in pastries, cakes, cheesecake, cookies, crackers or candies. Unless made at home, these foods are almost certain to contain fats that may elevate your cholesterol.

Most people don't connect chocolate with fat but a single ounce of milk chocolate contains 9.2 grams. And unless sold in healthfood stores, granola bars may contain partially-hydrogenated vegetable oils, as well as saturated fats or poly-unsaturated oils, and as many as a dozen sweeteners.

Oat bran muffins may sound healthy but the benefits of any oat bran they contain is usually more than offset by their high-fat content.

Another drawback is that most of these products are also made of fiber-less refined flour. Sweeteners are other refined carbohydrates liberally used in almost all bakery products. Whether sugar or honey, molasses, maple syrup, corn syrup or barley malt, none contains any fiber and all are capable of sending the blood sugar level soaring (only to have it plummet a short time later, leaving one feeling listless and depleted of energy).

If you want your cholesterol to stay down, and your health to stay up, you'd do well to avoid all commercially-made cakes, pastries, pies, cookies, doughnuts, candies, chocolate or sweeteners.

• Cholesterol Booster #8: Fried Foods, Potato Chips and Popcorn

In all of our three cholesterol-lowering plans, foods fried in saturated fats or polyunsaturated oils are strongly discouraged. Frying in monounsaturated oils like olive or canola oil is probably less harmful but it still multiplies fat consumption. Most fried foods in fast-food eateries and restaurants are loaded with undesirable fats.

French-fried potatoes or potato chips, or fried corn tortillas, rank among the fattiest foods eaten by Americans. A single ounce of potato chips can easily contain ten grams of fat and a one-ounce serving of commercially-prepared popcorn may also contain from five to eight grams of fat.

Like potatoes, popcorn is a healthful, low-fat food. That is, until we start adding fat, oil and salt to enhance the taste. The result is that some brands of microwave popcorn have five grams of fat per ounce with a fat content ranging from 56-76 per cent of calories. Some of this may be saturated fat. Air-popped or not, movie-theater popcorn frequently has up to eight grams of fat per one ounce serving.

• Cholesterol Booster #9: Commercial Dressings, Spreads and Sauces

The majority of regular salad dressings on supermarket shelves can transform a heart-healthy salad into an artery-clogging disaster. Some regular dressings are made of cheese, egg yolks and bacon and may get as much as 70 per cent of calories from fat.

One tablespoon of regular Italian dressing, for example, contains 9 grams of fat while blue cheese contains 7.8 and Russian 7.6. And because terms like "lite" or "reduced calorie" are not carefully monitored by the FDA, they can be almost meaningless. Some "lite" dressings have almost as much fat as regular dressings.

Regular mayonnaise is another high-fat food: one tablespoon contains two grams of saturated fat. Most "low-cal" or "low-fat" mayonnaise still contains half as much fat as regular, which is still an appreciable amount.

Commercial spreads, sauces, tomato sauces, whipped toppings and many supermarket brands of peanut butter (not *pure* peanut butter) may have a high content of saturated fat or partially-hydrogenated vegetable oil. Margarine is also often touted as preferable to butter but it is still high in partially-hydrogenated vegetable oils and contains significant amounts of saturated fat.

All shortening and vegetable shortening should also be eliminated and replaced with monounsaturated vegetable oils.

GUIDELINES FOR THE THREE CHOLESTEROL-LOWERING PLANS

With the exceptions previously noted, all of the foods mentioned as undesirable in Cholesterol Cutter #2 should be completely omitted from all three cholesterol-lowering plans in this book.

CHOLESTEROL CUTTER #3:

100 HEART-HEALTHY FOODS THAT HELP LOWER CHOLESTEROL

Low in fat and high in fiber, the 100 tasty complex carbohydrate foods listed below are the backbone of our three cholesterol-lowering plans. By eating these foods in place of the fat-laden foods identified in Cholesterol Cutter #2, your cholesterol level should commence a steady and prolonged decline.

Fruits

With the exception of avocados and dried fruits, all fresh fruits help in lowering cholesterol. Although healthful and nutritious, avocados and dried fruits should not be eaten until you have reached your cholesterol target level. Afterwards, they may be eaten sparingly.

Among the most common fruits are:

Apples	Papaya
Apricots	Peaches
Bananas	Pears
Berries, all types	Persimmons
Canteloupes	Pineapples
Cherries	Plums
Citrus, all types	Pomegranetes
Grapes	Rhubarb
Guavas	Star fruit
Kiwi fruit	Strawberries
Mangos	Watermelon
Melons, all types	

Vegetables

All fresh vegetables help in lowering cholesterol. Among the most readily-available vegetables are:

Asparagus	Chayote
Beets	Collards
Bok choy	Corn and hominy
Broccolli	Cucumbers
Brussels sprouts	Eggplant
Cabbage	Garlic
Cauliflower	Greens
Carrots	Green beans
Celery	Jicama

Kale
Kholrabi
Leeks
Lettuce
Mushrooms
Okra
Onions
Parsnips
Peppers, green and red

Potatoes
Rutabagas
Spinach
Squash, all types
Sweet potatoes, yams
Swiss chard
Tomatoes
Turnips
Watercress

Whole Grains

All whole grains help lower cholesterol. Healthfood stores and natural foods supermarkets generally have the best variety. Many are sold from open bins at low bulk prices. Among the most common are:

Amarynth
Barley
Buckwheat
Bulgar
Corn, cornmeal (unrefined)
Corn tortillas
Grits
Groats
Kasha
Millet
Muesli
Oats, oat bran, oatmeal
Wholegrain pasta
Rice, wild rice, rice bran
Rye, rye flour

Shredded wheat (and other sugar-free cereals made exclusively of whole grains and nothing else).
All sprouted grains and seeds
Triticale
Wheat, cracked wheat
Whole wheat flour
Whole grain breads and cereals (made exclusively of whole grains, or sprouted grains, and totally free of fats, oils, eggs or sweeteners).

Legumes

All types of beans and peas are high in fiber and vegetable protein and are powerful suppressors of LDL cholesterol.

Anasazi beans	Lentils
Azuki beans	Lima beans
Black beans	Navy beans
Black-eyed peas	Peas, all types
Butter beans	Peas, split
Garbanzo beans (chick peas)	Pinto beans
Great northern beans	Soy beans, tofu, tempeh
Kidney beans	

A Cholesterol-Lowering Taste Enhancer

Garlic deserves special mention because several studies have indicated that taking garlic over a period of weeks or months has lowered levels of fibrinogen in the bloodstream and has reduced the risk that a blood clot might set off a heart attack. Other experimenters have reported that garlic can lower cholesterol levels by approximately ten per cent. One problem is that garlic doesn't agree with everyone, and may cause stomach ulcers, anemia or allergic reactions.

However, these and other studies do provide a worthwhile indication and we suggest using one to two cloves of garlic a day as a food seasoner. For example, you might add two cloves to a soup or stew, and you could rub another squeezed clove over the bottom of your salad bowl. Odor-free garlic capsules may also be taken in supplements and in powder form. However, you are cautioned not to take garlic in amounts larger than is customarily used to season food.

140

A Real Nutrition Superstar

Bananas are another great heart-healthy food. A recent study by Dr. James E. Leklem, professor of foods and nutrition at the University of Oregon, found that many people with low levels of Vitamin B-6 also have higher cholesterol levels. Conversely, people given supplemental B-6 showed a reduced risk for heart disease.

In view of Dr. Leklem's research, it's worth noting that bananas are an excellent source of B-6. Five medium-sized bananas contain the equivalent of 45 per cent of the RDA for B-6. Bananas are also a good source of potassium, a deficiency of which has been associated with increased risk of stroke.

A study by Dr. Elizabeth Barrett-Connor of the University of California, San Diego, found that participants who ate the least amount of dietary potassium (1,950 mgs) were two-and-a-half times more likely to die of stroke than those who ate up to 2,600 mgs per day. During the 12-year study, 24 participants died of stroke and each had a below-average intake of potassium. Other studies have shown that people with a low potassium intake suffer more hypertension.

Avocados, although high in fat, also have a high content of both B-6 and potassium. Other complex carbohydrates high in potassium are beet greens, sweet potatoes, lima beans, canteloupes, acorn squash, potatoes, and spinach.

Guidelines for the Three Cholesterol-Lowering Plans

Regardless of which of our three plans you may be following, you may enjoy unlimited amounts of each of the foods listed in Cholesterol Cutter #3. Among the many healthy, fat-free foods are starchy foods such as beans, whole grain bread and pasta, potatoes, brown rice and other grains. These can be used to prepare a variety of filling and satisfying meals. Starch is actually quite low in calories yet its bulk helps to satisfy hunger as effectively as fat does.

CHOLESTEROL CUTTER #4:

LOWER YOUR CHOLESTEROL WITH SOLUBLE FIBER

Oat bran is all the rage these days for its cholesterol-lowering ability. Next year it may be rice bran or corn bran or psyllium seed. Each of these foods is high in soluble fiber.

When soluble fiber in food is digested and reaches the intestines, it binds with bile acids manufactured by the liver and gallbladder. To successfully emulsify and digest dietary fats, these bile acids must have a high cholesterol content. When soluble fiber binds with bile acids in the intestines, it prevents these bile acids from returning to the liver. Instead, they are excreted along with the fiber. This removes their cholesterol content from the body. It also forces the liver to draw down more cholesterol from the blood stream to replace the lost bile acid. In the process, the LDL cholesterol is lowered, usually without lowering HDL at all.

But before sprinkling oat bran on everything you eat, we need to put all the soluble fiber findings in their proper perspective.

Soluble fiber will very definitely help to lower cholesterol. But unless your total cholesterol is elevated to begin with— 240 mgs/dl or more—the decline may be rather modest. Exaggerated claims by some cereal manufacturers usually fail to state that the dramatic results they report occurred only in people whose cholesterol levels were alarmingly high to begin with.

An analysis of just about all of the studies done shows that, if your total cholesterol is 300 mgs/dl., a diet high in soluble fiber might drop it by as much as 20 per cent in a few weeks or months. But if your total cholesterol is 200 mgs/dl or less, soluble fiber may not take it down by more than three to five per cent. At lower cholesterol levels, soluble fiber has even less effect.

While soluble fiber isn't the magic elixir that some writers have claimed, it still remains an extremely heart-healthy food that each of us should eat every day. Even when our cholesterol level is already low, soluble fiber can help prevent it from rising back up again.

Without getting too involved in its biochemistry, suffice it to say that fiber comes in two basic types:

Soluble Fiber

Soft and malleable, and composed of pectins, gums and mucilage, soluble fiber dissolves in water and forms a gel when digested. Pectin, the substance that holds plant cells together, is capable of absorbing four times its own weight of cholesterol. Hence pectin is the primary agent which binds with bile acids to transport cholesterol out of the body.

Some researchers also claim that soluble fiber ferments in the colon, forming short-chain fatty acids which are absorbed into the portal vein and inhibit further synthesis of cholesterol in the liver.

Additionally, soluble fibers slow absorption of carbohydrates in the intestines, stabilizing blood sugar and insulin levels, and creating a feeling of fullness and satisfaction.

Insoluble Fiber

Insoluble fiber is coarse and spongy and does not dissolve in water. Consisting primarily of cellulose, it remains intact during digestion and absorbs large amounts of water. In turn, this creates soft, bulky stools that traverse the intestines at three to four times the speed of fat or protein. Many top researchers believe this prevents formation of carcinogens. Several large studies have confirmed that insoluble fiber consumption is associated with significantly lower rates of colon cancer, hemorrhoids, diverticulosis and constipation.

For optimal health, we need both types of fiber and most plant foods supply an abundance of each. By contrast, meat, fish, eggs, poultry and dairy foods contain very little fiber at all.

Virtually all complex carbohydrates contain adequate amounts of insoluble fiber, particularly wheat bran and wheat products, lentils and brown rice. And most beans, grains, fruits and vegetables contain soluble fiber.

Soluble Fiber Food Champions

Nonetheless, the *highest* levels of soluble fiber have been found in oat bran, cooked dried beans, corn bran, rice bran and oatmeal. Other foods high in soluble fiber include barley, baked potatoes, sweet potatoes and yams, broccoli, carrots, onions, leeks, asparagus, brussels sprouts and cooked corn. Crisp, crunchy apples are known for their high pectin content while figs, pears, oranges and bananas have more than their share.

Incidentally, the soluble fiber is in the fruit, not in the skin. Most of these foods also contain very adequate amounts of insoluble fiber.

Here is a brief look at some soluble fiber champs.

- Oat Bran is the ground inner husk of the oat grain and it contains more soluble fiber than almost any other food. One cup has a total fiber content exceeding five grams, of which 2.2 grams is soluble fiber. According to a California study, eating half a cup of oat bran per day for four weeks reduced cholesterol levels 5.3 per cent in the average person.
- Corn Bran. Several studies have shown that corn bran is as effective at lowering cholesterol as oat bran. It can be used as a substitute for cornmeal when making pancakes or quick breads.
- Rice Bran is the husk of the rice kernel. In animal studies, it has reportedly lowered cholesterol by 25 per cent. It makes a tasty hot cereal or can be added to muffins or yeast breads.
- Oatmeal is the flattened flake of the whole oat grain. A one-ounce serving contains 1.5 ounces of soluble fiber. In several studies, oatmeal has lowered cholesterol by the same amount as oat bran.
- Psyllium husks are a form of soluble fiber found in some breakfast cereals and in a bulk-forming laxative better known as Metamucil. A 1989 study at the University of Minnesota found that one teaspoon per day for 12 weeks dropped total cholesterol by an average 15 per cent in people with elevated cholesterol. In another group with more normal levels, eight weeks on psyllium reduced their LDL

levels by an average 8.2 per cent while their HDL was unaffected. Since psyllium also acts as a laxative, one must be careful of over consumption.

How Much Soluble Fiber Do We Need?

Most nutritionists recommend eating a bowl of oatmeal, a cup of cooked oat bran, a cup of cooked dry beans, or three oat bran muffins free of eggs, sugar, or oil each day. The best way to ensure getting enough fiber is to eat a bowl of oatmeal or cooked oat bran as a breakfast cereal, and to have half a cup of cooked dry beans at a later meal.

For a quick meal of beans, you could heat up one eight-ounce can of vegetarian-style baked beans sold in supermarkets. In one study, eating a can of baked beans daily for several weeks reduced cholesterol by 13 per cent in a group of people whose total cholesterol averaged 200 mgs/dl. Health food stores have an abundance of prepared bean dishes such as vegetarian chili or lentil soup.

Both the AHA and the NCI have recommended increasing total fiber intake from the meagre 10.5 grams eaten daily by the average American to 20-30 grams or more. Many experts believe we should consume 30-35 grams of fiber and some recommend 40 or more. The average Chinese eats 34 grams per day.

Some dieticians have expressed concern that eating more than 35 grams daily could compromise mineral absorption. But in practice, no association has ever been found, and some people in China consume 70 grams of fiber a day without affecting their mineral status.

Ease Your Way Into a High Fiber Diet.

Nevertheless, in switching to a high fiber diet, several cautions should be observed.

1. During your initial cholesterol test (see Chapter 2), you should check with your doctor to ensure that it is okay for you to eat a high fiber diet. If you have a bowel disorder or kidney disease, or if you could possibly develop a blocked bowel, or have had recent surgery, you need medical clearance before increasing dietary fiber.

2. Increase fiber gradually or you may experience gas, flatulence or bloating. To minimize gas, soak all legumes before cooking, discard the soaking water, and avoid mixing beans with cabbage family vegetables. Most high fiber foods also require more chewing than other foods.

3. Since fiber sponges up water from the intestines, drink at least 6-8 glasses of water daily.

Most healthy people can make the transition to eating 30 grams or more of fiber daily in just a short time.

Oat Bran Doughnuts

From muffins to doughnuts, bagels, bread and breakfast cereals, processors are putting oat bran into dozens of commercial foods. Oftentimes, the amount is too small to be effective. And when there is enough oat bran to do any good, its benefits are frequently offset by a high dose of oil, sugar, or egg yolk. So check all labels carefully for saturated fat, poly-unsaturated oils, partially-hydrogenated vegetable oils, or eggs. And unless oat bran is listed among the first three ingredients, there usually isn't enough to be of any benefit.

147

For those unable to digest fiber, supplements may help to lower cholesterol and reduce the risk of colon cancer. However, they should be used only when dietary fiber cannot be eaten. The best supplements are probably those made of coarse, compressed wheat bran, soy fiber or ground psyllium husks. Follow the manufacturer's instructions. And don't forget that it's quite possible to overdose on fiber supplements.

GUIDELINES FOR THE THREE CHOLESTEROL-LOWERING PLANS

Regardless of which plan you are following, let your body be your guide and eat the amount of dietary fiber that feels right for you. Just by selecting a variety of the foods listed in Cholesterol Cutter #3, you will be eating far more fiber— both soluble and insoluble—than the average American.

CHOLESTEROL CUTTER #5:

DON'T LET DECEPTIVE LABELS SABOTAGE YOUR CHOLESTEROL

Nutritional labels, originally placed on foods to reveal their contents, have become a means of disguising and distorting the levels of total fat and saturated fat in hundreds of lines of packaged foods.

A label may truthfully proclaim "no cholesterol." In fact, no plant-based food has any cholesterol at all. Yet that same food can be so high in saturated fat, or in total fat, that it can send your cholesterol level skyward. For example, pure peanut butter contains no cholesterol yet is 50 per cent fat (of which one-eighth is saturated). And polyunsaturated oils, also cholesterol-free, are 100 per cent fat.

All labels on meat and poultry are regulated by the USDA while those on other foods are supervised by the FDA. But enforcement is often lax. The result is that manufacturers have learned to disguise their ingredients in a variety of sneaky terms.

Words like monoglycerides, diglycerides or triglycerides may all be used on labels as synonyms for fat, as are terms like butterfat, whole milk solids, shortening or schmaltz (poultry fat). Any of these terms could also refer to saturated fat.

Equally misleading are such ambiguous terms as "new," "real," "natural," "health food," "high fiber," or "contains no artificial anything"—all widely used on food packages and labels. To make them all the more difficult to decipher, nutritional labels are frequently printed in minuscule type on transparent paper, or are otherwise made as difficult as possible to read. While shopping in a health food store isn't an ironclad guarantee of finding safe packaged foods, it certainly does multiply the odds in your favor.

Misleading Labels

On meat or poultry, "Lite" or "Light" must signify that a food contains 25 per cent less fat, sodium, breading or calories than the regular version. "Low fat" dairy products must not contain more than .5 to two per cent fat by weight. And "reduced calorie" foods must have one-third fewer calories than regular versions.

These exceptions apart, terms like "low cal" or "low fat" have few standards. "Light" can refer to a food's light color or its light texture or to its being light in calories. Despite all this, many "light" or "low cal" foods may still be high in fat. Some "light" frozen dinners, for example, derive 30-42 per cent of calories from fat and many still feature regular beef or cheese.

A "cholesterol-free" label signifies that a food contains less than two mgs of cholesterol per serving. "Low cholesterol" means it has less than 20 mgs per serving. And "cholesterol-reduced" means that a food has 75 per cent less cholesterol than the regular product.

Most nutritional labels break down contents under three headings. One, the "Percentage of U.S. RDAs"—a long list of vitamins and minerals meant to impress purchasers—can be disregarded here. Under "Nutritional Information Per Serving" is given the serving size together with the weight in grams of protein, carbohydrates and fat. The more reputable manufacturers, especially those whose products are sold in health food stores, may also break down total fat into the weight in grams of saturated and poly-unsaturated fats. Some also quote the percentage of calories from fat and the weight, in milligrams, of cholesterol.

How Labels Camouflage Fat

Always bear in mind that the fat content is more important than the cholesterol content and that the key to total fat content is the percentage of calories derived from fat. Where only the grams of total fat and the number of calories per serving are given, the percentage of calories derived from fat can easily be calculated by using the formula quoted earlier in this chapter under "How To Calculate The Fat Content of Any Processed Food" (see page 120).

Regardless of serving size, this formula will give you the real fat content of any food. Whether by intent or merely to confuse the public, serving sizes are often given in varying amounts—from two-thirds of a cupful to two tablespoons, from two-thirds of an ounce to four-fifths of an ounce, or typically, one-and-a-quarter ounces. One package just examined quoted serving size as one ounce while each slice actually weighed three-fourths of an ounce. Such inconsistencies can easily throw off the uninformed consumer. However, by using our formula for finding the percentage of calories from fat, serving size can be ignored.

The other key to fat content is the list of ingredients. All labels list ingredients in descending order of weight (not volume). Any food that lists a fat, oil or egg yolk in the first three or four ingredients should be suspect.

A quick perusal of the labels just described will reveal, for instance, how many "low cal" cheeses have the same fat content as regular cheese.

Staying Afloat in a Nutritional Quicksand

Your trusty calculator can also save you from being duped by claims such as "80 per cent fat-free" or "20 per cent fat." These percentages, which appear on one brand of "lite" bologna, refer to weight. They do not refer to the percentage of calories from fat—which nutritionists consider the only meaningful way of measuring fat content.

Since fat supplies nine calories per gram, versus only four calories per gram of carbohydrate or protein, it follows that, in this particular case,

$$20 \text{ per cent} \times 9 = 180$$
$$80 \text{ per cent} \times 4 = 320$$
$$100 \text{ per cent} = 500$$

If 500 = 100 per cent, then 180 = 36 per cent—meaning that 36 per cent of this "lite" luncheon meat's calories is derived from fat, not the mere 20 per cent implied on the label.

You should be particularly careful of such labels on processed meats. Remember that all label percentages refer to weight. On a calorie basis, ham labeled "95 per cent fat-free" still derives 11 or more per cent of calories from fat. While such meats represent a big improvement over the regular version, they still have appreciably more than the five percent of fat implied by the label.

When buying processed poultry, look for the words "breast meat," "meat" or "skinless" on the label. But if the label bears only the words "breast" or "thighs" without referring to "meat" or "skinless," the product *may* contain appreciable amounts of skin. As you may recall, half the fat in a chicken is in the skin. A processed chicken product containing skin may have as much fat as an equal amount of hamburger.

The Refined Carbohydrate Snare

Sugar is often hidden on labels under names ending in "-ose." For instance, sugar may be described as dextrose, glucose, sucrose, fructose or maltose. Other forms of sugar appear on labels as cane sugar, maple sugar, brown sugar, barley malt, malted barley, sorbitol, sorghum molasses, rice syrup, raw sugar, corn syrup, cane sugar, honey or grape sweetener. All are refined carbohydrates that can send your blood sugar level soaring and, indirectly, have a less-than-desirable effect on your cholesterol.

Another nutritional snare is a bread package bearing the announcement, "Made with 100% Pure Whole Wheat

Flour." Yet the first item on the ingredient list is "enriched wheat flour"—meaning white flour—while the whole grain flour is the third or fourth ingredient (and is frequently followed by another refined carbohydrate such as high fructose corn syrup and/or corn syrup).

As the package correctly claims, the loaf is made *with* 100 per cent whole wheat flour. But it's not 100 per cent whole wheat flour, as the label implies. Instead of the beneficial whole grain you expected, you're getting twice as much refined carbohydrate and half as much fiber. Although some supermarkets do stock genuine fat-free, whole grain breads, in many cities the only place to find a wholesome bread is at a health food store. Breads without labels are a wildcard that is best avoided.

Although new labelling proposals are constantly under review by the FDA, it may be years before any real reforms appear. Meanwhile, the only way to avoid becoming a heart disease statistic is to become adept at reading the current labels.

CHOLESTEROL CUTTER #6:

TEN WAYS TO EAT LEAN AND CLEAN

Here are ten simple ways to keep saturated fat and cholesterol out of your diet.

• Anti-Cholesterol Step #1: Healthful Foods to Temporarily Avoid

Nuts, seeds, olives and avocados are among the most healthful of natural foods. Yet many varieties are high in fat,

153

including saturated fat. Half a cup of cashews contains 52 grams of fat while a cup of Brazil nuts has 46.5 grams. Sunflower and other seeds also contain appreciable amounts of fat.

We'd suggest omitting all nuts, seeds, avocados and olives until your total and LDL cholesterols have dropped to their target levels. After that, you can begin to eat sparingly of avocados, olives and seeds and some of the less fatty nuts.

Among the fattiest nuts are coconuts, macadamias, Brazils, cashews, filberts, walnuts, almonds, pistachios and pecans. Most nuts get 65-85 per cent of calories from fat. To include even a few nuts in your diet can easily run up your daily total of fat calories by ten per cent.

Peanuts are almost as high in fat as are sunflower, sesame and pumpkin seeds. Avocados and olives also derive about 80 per cent of calories from fat (even though most *is* unsaturated). We'd also temporarily avoid peanut butter and any other nut butters or nut oils. Even though low in saturated fat, they still get 50 per cent or more of calories from fat.

Other nutritious foods like tofu and tempeh can also be surprisingly high in fat. They, too, should be eaten sparingly, and then only after reaching your cholesterol target level. Chestnuts have the lowest fat content of any nut.

• Anti-Cholesterol Step #2: Don't Ruin Healthy Foods by Adding Fat

A medium-sized baked potato has almost no fat. But slathering it with 4 tablespoons of sour cream adds more saturated fat than there is in a small steak. Likewise, a cup of oatmeal has only .4 grams of fat. But add a pat of butter and one-third cup of whole milk, and you end up with 4.6 grams of fat—equivalent to eating two eggs.

Often we start out right by choosing foods low in fat and high in fiber. But it's what we put on them before eating that makes them high risk. When eating the low-cholesterol way, a baked potato means exactly that. It doesn't mean a potato smothered in butter or cream. And a slice of bread doesn't mean bread covered with butter or margarine or anything else.

Instead of fat-laden toppings and spreads, use plain nonfat yogurt on baked potatoes. Better still are salsa or mustard or tasty spices like celery seed, thyme, rosemary, marjoram or a mixed herb seasoning.

• Anti-Cholesterol Step #3: Avoid the Convenience Food Trap

The majority of prepared, processed, canned or packaged supermarket foods are loaded with fats, calories and salt. Even foods labeled "lite" offer only a token reduction. For example, bread crumb mixes are notoriously high in fat, some of which may be saturated. Most bouillon cubes can also sabotage your fat-reduction plans. With few exceptions, healthful food just isn't sold in packages, boxes, bottles or cans. It's all located in the produce section of your supermarket and it's sold by the pound or by the bunch or dozen.

To lower your cholesterol, replace as much frozen, canned and processed foods as you can with primary foods. That means fresh, unfragmented foods in the same unchanged state in which they grew in nature: fruits fresh off the tree, vegetables fresh from the field, and grains that have never been refined. The more processed a food, the less fiber and the more added fat and sugar it is likely to have.

Half the food eaten in America is mass-produced, convenience food—liberally coated with fat and salt and all ready to pop in the oven or microwave. If you possibly can, avoid falling for this cholesterol trap. Instead, try to shop twice a week and buy more fresh, complex carbohydrate foods. And take an extra half hour two or three times a week to prepare fresh, whole foods.

If you simply don't have time to cook whole foods every night, consider making a large pot of vegetable stew, soup or steamed vegetables—or any other low-fat, high fiber dish—in a quantity sufficient to last for three days. Cook it on Sunday, then refrigerate. This way, you're guaranteed a healthy dinner on Monday and Tuesday. Freezing soups or stews for the next week—or month—is another possibility.

• Anti-Cholesterol Step #4: Eat More Raw Fruits and Vegetables

Few Americans have ever eaten a real vegetable salad. Most of us think of a salad as a few bits of lettuce, tomato and cucumber served as a side dish in a small bowl.

Instead, try this. Chop up and mix together one head of leaf lettuce (avoid iceberg if possible which has practically no nutritional value), one cucumber, one red or green pepper, three grated carrots, one packet of alfalfa or mixed sprouts, eight green onions, some chopped greens, half a chopped jicama, four medium-sized tomatoes, and some finely chopped broccoli flowerets or cauliflower. Other vegetables, such as radishes or watercress, can be added in season. Once you've reached your cholesterol target level, you can include a chopped-up avocado. For a dressing, consider plain, nonfat yogurt or one of the fat-free commercial dressings.

Instead of pouring olive oil on to a salad, thin it first with a mild vinegar such as "balsamic"—and keep the olive oil to a minimum. One teaspoon of olive oil and two teaspoons of balsamic vinegar will nicely flavor one salad. You can impart still more flavor by adding tasty spices like parsley, cilantro, basil, dill or arugula, or even Belgian endive or mustard greens. You can also bulk up salads by adding cooked green beans, kidney or garbanzo beans. Canned beans will do in a pinch.

A salad this noble is a meal in itself. To help dispel the concept of meat-centered meals, fill a large bowl with this healthful salad and serve it as the main course. Add to the fun by eating it with chopsticks. Refrigerated, a salad this size should last 3 days.

While you're at it, fix a fresh fruit salad for dessert. Mix together four or five different fresh fruits and serve as is or topped with plain, nonfat yogurt. The more plant-based foods you can work into your diet, the less room there is for cholesterol-promoting foods of animal origin.

• Anti-Cholesterol Step #5: Eat Less Salt

Since salt may contribute to arterial plaque, intake should be limited to a maximum of one-fourth of a teaspoon per day from all sources. People with hypertension should not exceed one-fifth of a teaspoon per day. And for optimal health, two pinches a day would be plenty. There's little need to add salt to any recipe, and low sodium varieties of many processed foods are now available.

• Anti-Cholesterol Step #6: Never Snack on Junk Food

Research has revealed that most of what we call a "sweet tooth" is actually a "fat tooth." Under scrutiny, the two most popular sweet snacks—ice cream and candy bars—turn out to be not only high in sugar but also high in fats. Cakes and muffins are just as bad. A single croissant has 12 grams of fat and a typical muffin has ten.

Instead of driving up your cholesterol by snacking on food of dubious benefit, try eating an apple, orange, pear or banana, or some seedless grapes. Or try a bowl of strawberries, or a sliced persimon mixed with a sliced banana and smothered in plain, nonfat yogurt. You can also cut apple or pear wedges for snacks, wedges of cauliflower or carrots, and serve with slices of lemon. Try freezing a peeled banana—or a peach or seedless grapes or a slice of melon—in the freezing compartment of your refrigerator. A frozen banana makes a wonderful substitute for ice cream while other frozen fruit snacks provide a unique taste experience.

Snacking on oranges is a splendid way to get artery-clearing Vitamin C. A recent study by Dr. Ishwalal Jialal, professor of clinical nutrition at the University of Texas Southwest Medical Center, found that just 60 mgs of Vitamin C daily dramatically slowed build-up of cholesterol plaque in arteries. One medium-sized orange daily supplies the needed amount of Vitamin C. But an extra orange or two won't hurt. While you could obtain the Vitamin C from squeezed orange juice, eating the fruit gives you more fiber—a fact that applies as well to all other fruits and vegetables.

Surprisingly, fig newtons or whole wheat fig bars, or rice cakes, matzo or pretzels are all relatively low in fat and make tasty and wholesome snacks. But the best all-around snack is probably plain, air-popped popcorn. Flavor with any herb or spice like curry, garlic or chili powder.

• Anti-Cholesterol Step #7: Avoid the High Cholesterol Aisles in Your Supermarket

To shop lean and clean, pass up the cholesterol aisles and head straight for the produce section of your supermarket, a one-stop shop that literally sells protection from high cholesterol as well as from heart disease, stroke, cancer, diabetes, osteoporosis and kidney disease.

Except for skim milk and plain, nonfat yogurt, stay away from the dairy cases and the deli section. Apart from a few whole grains and dried beans, aisle after aisle in the typical supermarket is lined with meat, eggs and dairy foods plus hundreds of boxed and packaged foods that most of us would be better off without.

Never shop on an empty stomach and carry a calculator with the fat calories formula taped to it. If you buy any extras, make sure they are complex carbohydrates.

• Anti-Cholesterol Step #8: Buy Only Heart-Smart Dairy Foods

Skim milk, or powdered skim milk, is by far the safest type of milk to drink. By comparison, even one per cent fat milk gets 18 per cent of calories from fat. Yet skim milk has the same calcium and protein content as whole milk. Skim milk buttermilk also has the same low-fat content as skim milk and can be safely used in baked goods or pancakes.

The best substitute for cream cheese is undoubtedly yogurt cheese (see Cholesterol Cutter #8). Soy-based cheese substitutes are also okay. Where available, sapsago or goat milk cheeses are low in fat and both can be crumbled over pasta

159

dishes. Goat milk cheese has only one gram of fat per ounce. The safest cottage cheeses are those made with the driest curds. Nonfat cottage cheese is now available.

Plain nonfat yogurt is undoubtedly one of few genuinely heart-healthy dairy products. Which explains why some food manufacturers have jumped on the yogurt bandwagon by coating fatty foods with yogurt, then claiming them as healthy, low-fat foods.

Frozen or whipped yogurt may be loaded with fat or sugar. Be on the alert, too, for yogurt look-alikes designed to taste like yogurt but which contain little or no real yogurt at all. Other yogurt-coated snacks may be just plain candy loaded with fat and sugar. Up to one-fifth of some frozen yogurts are laced with sugar, milk and stabilizers. (Sugar overload aside, however, low-fat frozen yogurt usually has about one-eighth the fat content of ice cream, to which it is infinitely preferable.)

You'll find most of these yogurt deceptions carried in the frozen food cases in your supermarket. Hence it makes sense to buy yogurt only in the dairy cases. Anything but plain, nonfat yogurt is suspect. (We assume you know that fruit-flavored yogurt usually contains an excess of sugar and additives.)

A very recent development, not available everywhere yet, is fat-free cheddar, American and mozzarella cheeses, claimed to have a fat content of zero. Some nutritionists also recommend lite ricotta cheese.

• Anti-Cholesterol Step #9: Make Your Carbohydrates Complex

It's worth knowing that a low-fat diet in which only refined carbohydrates are eaten is not nearly as effective as a diet rich in complex carbohydrates. The soluble fiber in these plant foods actully soaks up the cholesterol and fat in your diet and speeds it to the intestines where it is excreted from your body.

• Anti-Cholesterol Step #10: Farewell to Fat in the Meat Department

If you continue to buy beef, you'll want to know that tenderloin, round and flank cuts are usually leanest. Instead of "choice" or "prime" beef or marbled cuts, look for "select" grades with the least visible fat. Although they're far from fat-free, "extra-lean" grades of beef, pork or lamb are preferable. The lowest-fat cuts are: beef—eye of round and top round; lamb—shank or leg; pork—tenderloin.

The USDA defines "lean" meat as having no more than ten per cent of fat by weight (21 per cent in terms of fat calories) and "extra lean" as having no more than five per cent (10.5 per cent in fat calories). One problem has been that, as this was written, not all states were conforming to these standards and the average fat content of "lean" ground beef nationwide was 21 per cent by weight while "extra lean" was 17 per cent by weight.

Special range-bred, low-fat beef is being raised in South Dakota and, perhaps, elsewhere by now, in which only ten per cent of calories are from fat while it has less than half the saturated fat content of choice beef.

Also, if you continue to buy luncheon meat, at least have it sliced "extra-thin"—or buy it in packages marked "extra-thin." Skinless chicken, turkey or very low-fat ham are probably the safest luncheon meats with sliced turkey breast ranking among the leanest of all deli items.

Yet wild game still remains the safest meat. Venison, buffalo or wild turkey (but not wild duck or goose) are all exceptionally low in fat. Turkey breast has the lowest fat content of any domestic poultry meat, and rabbit is also low in fat.

The safest seafoods appear to be clams, mussels, oysters and crab while squid has more cholesterol and saturated fat. Shrimp, scallops and lobster come somewhere in between. Again, water-packed canned fish or seafood has considerably less fat than the same foods packed in oil. Among the least fatty fish are sole and flounder.

Regardless of how low their fat content, all animal-based foods are still high in animal protein. Far safer are plant-based meat substitutes, such as plain tofu or tempeh, tofu hot dogs, soy or grain-based burgers, and seitan—a meat look-alike made out of wheat gluten. Soy products are also available to replace cheese while soy-based desserts are far healthier than ice cream.

A final tip for those with dentures. High-fiber foods such as raw fruits and vegetables, require more chewing and mastication than refined carbohydrates or other soft foods. If you have trouble chewing fiber, make your vegetables into soups and stews and cut fresh fruits into very small pieces.

GUIDELINES FOR THE THREE CHOLESTEROL-LOWERING PLANS

The Easy-Does-It Plan permits up to three ounces of very lean meat to be eaten daily. So make sure any meat you eat really is exceptionally lean, and avoid using any luncheon meat but skinless turkey, chicken or very low-fat ham. A three-ounce serving of meat is equal in size to a pack of playing cards.

CHOLESTEROL CUTTER #7:

COOKING WITHOUT CHOLESTEROL

To lower their cholesterol, thousands of Americans have embarked on a new culinary lifestyle. Their meals have a new look. Instead of focusing on a centerpiece of meat or poultry, succulent vegetables, beans and grains fill their plates. If meat, poultry or fish is included at all, it's just a few pieces dotted around the edge of the plate as a condiment.

Cooking the healthful, low-cholesterol way means rethinking what a plate of food looks like. Far from tasting bland or drab, plant-based recipes can provide peak experiences in cooking taste and enjoyment. You don't have to live on sprouts or carrots. All the rich, subtle flavors and pungent seasonings of exotic Third World countries are yours to enjoy.

From countries where the average cholesterol level is far lower than ours come hundreds of exciting, heart-healthy recipes. To sample the pastas of Italy, the curries of south India, or the bouillabaisse of Provence, will quickly convince you that "gourmet cooking" *is* compatible with low cholesterol. From the great culinary traditions of China, Japan and India you can draw on dozens of tasty, grain-based dishes, virtually every one free of saturated fat and cholesterol.

In Mediterranean countries, where olive oil adds luster to almost every food, people traditionally eat only small, lean portions of meat and few, if any, dairy foods. Which probably explains why the people of the Greek island of Crete turned out to be the most heart-healthy in the landmark Seven Countries Study.

163

Superlean Cookware

Since you have complete control over all ingredients, cooking at home is far safer than eating out. A good way to begin is to replace all deep fryers and traditional frying pans with the no-stick skillets sold in department stores. (It's also possible to fry without fat in a cast-iron skillet provided it is first "seasoned" by being used for conventional frying several times. This seals the pores, after which it must never come into contact with water. To clean, you wipe it with a paper towel.)

A pressure cooker will cook beans or rice in 15-25 minutes and soup in under 20 minutes. A steamer is almost essential. And a slow crock pot will cook grains or beans without burning while you're out shopping or exercising; or it will cook soybeans overnight while you sleep. For roasting chicken, consider using a vertical poultry-roasting rack which holds the bird upright in the oven while fat drips down into a pan. This prevents a pan-cooked bird from stewing in its own pool of melted fat. Alternatively, you can still cook a bird in a pan and keep it out of the fat by raising it on a cookie rack.

The small size of this book prevents us from giving more than a brief selection of our favorite recipes (see CC#8). However, virtually every library has a shelf of vegetarian and oriental or macrobiotic cookbooks filled with healthful recipes.

Vegetarian Doesn't Always Mean Low Fat

Unfortunately, not all vegetarian cookbooks are filled with healthful recipes. When it comes to cholesterol, the word vegetarian has more than one meaning.

Many ethical vegetarians are lacto-ovo, meaning they eat dairy foods and eggs. Others may be lacto or ovo-vegetarians. Since many of their recipes lean heavily on butter, oil, cheese or eggs, lacto or ovo-vegetarians tend to consume more saturated fat and cholesterol than do many people who eat meat or skinless poultry.

A total vegetarian, or vegan, eats only fruits, vegetables, whole grains, legumes, nuts and seeds—in other words, a genuine plant-based diet. Thus the most healthful recipes are those you will find in vegan or macrobiotic cookbooks.

Slash the Fat Across the Board

Since lacto-ovo vegetarians avoid only flesh foods, it's hardly surprising that many of their recipes call for dangerously high amounts of oil, fat or eggs. Like those in standard cookbooks, they pile on far more butter, margarine and poly-unsaturated oils than are really needed.

As a result we have found that, almost invariably, we can slash *at least two-thirds* of the fat and oil in any recipe without really noticing the difference. Additionally, egg whites can replace egg yolks. When fat is really essential, use olive or canola oils.

By changing the way we cook, we can plan every meal as a healthful, low-fat repast. So steam, poach, bake, boil or broil but *never* fry in fat or oil. Foods that are relatively low-fat like chicken, fish or potatoes can become supercharged with fat while frying. A single helping of fried chicken often has twice the fat as an equal-sized portion of marbled sirloin steak.

Frying is doubly dangerous because fats are chemically fragile when heated to frying temperatures, and polyunsaturated fats in particular can become so oxidized that they release free radicals. When digested, these reactive agents can injure coronary artery walls, create arterial plaque and increase risk of cancer. Also, never cook in hot butter or margarine. Nor are corn and soy oils recommended for any type of cooking, including baking. The safest cooking oils are olive or canola oil.

Olive oil comes in several varieties. "Extra virgin" has a delicate flavor and contains a maximum of one per cent of free oleic acid. "Fine virgin" is similar but may have up to 1.5 per cent of free oleic. "Semi-fine" or "ordinary" virgin has a pleasant flavor and not more than three per cent of free oleic acid. "Light" olive oil has the same fat and calorie content as regular olive oil but is processed to give it a milder flavor. No one variety appears to offer any appreciable health benefit over the others.

By the way, here's how to make a filling non-fat substitute for French fries. Cut a scrubbed baking potato into wedges. Brush the wedges lightly with olive oil (one teaspoon will do it). Then simply bake them at 450° on a cookie sheet for about 30 minutes. Delicious! You can also make your own fat-free tortilla chips by cutting up some corn tortillas and baking them in the same way without any oil at all.

Making Eggs Safe to Eat

Egg yolks are a no-no in low-cholesterol cooking. Each yolk contains 5.6 grams of fat and 213 mgs of cholesterol. By comparison, each egg white has barely a trace of fat, no cholesterol and 3.3 grams of whole protein.

Since three egg whites are permitted daily in each of our cholesterol-lowering plans, here is how to separate them.

Break the center of an egg on the rim of a saucepan or bowl. Draw the two halves slowly apart and catch the yolk in one half. As you gently pass the yolk back and forth, from one half to the other, allow the white to drain into the pan or bowl. Should any yolk fall into the white, scoop it out.

Egg whites can be used in cooking wherever eggs are called for. Use several to make an omelette, then put some tomatoes or onions on top in place of the yolk. Alternatively, scramble four egg whites with one yolk and split it with another person—for a total of only 107 mgs of cholesterol each—versus the 426 mgs of two whole eggs.

Watch That Chicken Skin

Never add any oil or fat to a chicken to moisten the meat or buy a pre-basted bird.

Home-made breaded chicken patties have less than half the fat content of commercial varieties. To make low-fat patties, use a boneless, skinless chicken. Dust it with flour or cornmeal. Then fry it in a no-stick skillet that has been lightly sprayed with nonfat, vegetable spray. For added flavor, add herbs and spices to the flour or cornmeal coating.

Low-fat fish fillets of haddock, pollack, halibut, sole or flounder can be made in the same way.

Low Fat Creams and Cheeses That Taste Terrific

Yogurt cheese is a healthy, nonfat substitute for cream cheese or sour cream. To make it, line a large filter or strainer with three layers of cheesecloth or a coffee filter. (In a pinch, you could use paper towels.) Place 4 cups (one quart) of plain, nonfat yogurt inside, stand in a bowl, refrigerate, and allow to drain overnight. After the whey drains off, you'll have 1½-2 cups of smooth, creamy yogurt cheese inside. Each cup has 135 calories and no fat while regular cream cheese has 400 calories and 39 grams of fat.

Yogurt cheese is delicious on baked potatoes or as a topping for fresh fruit, waffles or pancakes. It can also be spread on bread, toast or bagels or used as a dip for crisp, raw vegetables.

One tip: check that your brand of nonfat yogurt is free of emulsifiers and stabilizers that prevent the whey from draining out. To check, scoop a depression in a carton of yogurt and allow to stand for 20 minutes. If the depression fills with liquid, your brand should be okay.

Although plain, nonfat yogurt by itself makes a satisfactory substitute for sour cream, a richer, thicker version can be made like this. Purée some light ricotta or low-fat or nonfat cottage cheese. Mix in an equal amount of plain, nonfat yogurt. The result so closely resembles sour cream that most people have difficulty telling the difference. Another good place to use plain, nonfat yogurt, or skim milk buttermilk is to replace the egg, oil or cream in home-made salad dressings (Caesar, French or Thousand Island).

Pass the Grains

Although unfamiliar to most Americans, millet, wheat and barley are delicious grains to cook and eat with vegetables and beans. To cook, simply add two-and-one-half cups of water to one cup of grain and cook in a crock pot. Any grain can be cooked in the same way. Incidentally, to keep fresh vegetables crisp, wrap in a paper towel and insert into a plastic bag before refrigerating.

Judiciously-chosen herbs and spices can more than replace

all the taste that salt, fat, mayonnaise and dressings provide in most foods. Almost all health food stores, natural foods stores, and supermarkets stock a variety of tasty herbs including basil, chili powder, chives, cilantro, curry powder, dill, garlic, oregano, paprika, pepper, rosemary and thyme.

GUIDELINES FOR THE THREE CHOLESTEROL-LOWERING PLANS

Each day, we should try to eat up to seven servings of vegetables; four of fresh, whole fruit; five of whole grain cereals including bread, cooked grains or pasta; and one of legumes like peas or beans. An optional additional serving of three egg whites would add about ten grams of whole protein with zero fat or cholesterol.

Fiberpack Your Breakfast and Lunch

Breakfast is the best meal for obtaining fiber. Typically, one could eat a bowl of oatmeal, or any other whole grain cereal, sprinkled with a generous topping of fresh fruits, such as cut-up apple, canteloupe, banana and and/or pineapple. Canned pineapple chunks can be used if fresh is not available. Try to avoid mixing citrus with sweet fruits. Any fresh fruit in season can be used including watermelon.

Some of your plain, nonfat yogurt allowance could be used as a topping. By rotating the grains and fruits, this same breakfast combination is always welcome and refreshing.

Soup and salad; vegetable chili with beans; black beans with rice and corn tortillas; a vegetable stew; eggplant and vegetables with baked potato; a split pea or lentil soup with whole grain bread; or a whole grain pita pocket stuffed with salad vegetables, are just a few of scores of low-fat lunch possibilities.

For dinner entrées, we suggest turning to Cholesterol Cutter #8.

Whatever you choose to eat, try to learn to enjoy a meal because it benefits your health. As you get into the low-cholesterol way of eating and cooking, you'll discover that the healthier the meal, the more you'll enjoy it.

CHOLESTEROL CUTTER #8:

TWELVE FAVORITE FAT-FREE RECIPES

Experience shows that the average family has a repertoire of only 10-12 recipes which they rotate for dinner night after night. If any of your favorite recipes are high in fat, consider substituting one of the twelve low-fat entrees described below. All are free of fats or oils and consist entirely of plant-based foods.

These recipes are given primarily as proof that tasty, satisfying meals are possible without using meat, dairy foods, butter, egg yolks, oils or fats. A tremendous variety of heart-friendly dishes is possible by steaming or baking vegetables together with tasty herbs and serving them with various combinations of rice, millet or barley. Again, the variety of vegetable soups and stews is almost endless.

Carrot Casserole   Serves Four

2½ cups *finely diced carrots*

2 *egg whites, lightly beaten*

½ cup water

1 *medium onion, finely chopped*

1 *tablespoon honey*

¼ cup cornmeal

2 *tablespoons fresh dill weed (or 1 tablespoon dried)*

¼ cup sunflower seeds

salt

Place the carrots, onions and water, together with two pinches of salt, in a saucepan. Bring to a boil, then allow to simmer for 20 minutes until the carrots are just tender. Meanwhile, pre-heat the oven to 350°. Into the saucepan stir the sunflower seeds, dill, honey, egg whites and cornmeal. Mix well. Lightly oil a baking dish with nonfat vegetable spray. Pour the contents of the saucepan into the baking dish. Bake for 15 minutes. Serve alone or with a side dish of rice, barley or millet.

Eggplant Casserole   Serves Six

2 green or red bell
  peppers
6 medium zucchini
4 large tomatoes
2 large onions
1 medium eggplant
1 clove of garlic
½ cup chopped parsley
1 teaspoon low-sodium
  soy sauce
1 teaspoon crushed
  oregano

Slice the onions; cut the tomatoes into chunks; cut the eggplant into ½-inch cubes; slice the zucchini into ½-inch thick slices; and cut the bell peppers into ½-inch squares.

Mix together all the ingredients and place in a six-quart casserole and cover. Bake at 350° for 90 minutes. During the first 60 minutes, baste with the vegetable juices that appear during baking. After baking 90 minutes, remove the cover and bake an additional 30 minutes.

Indian Cauliflower and Rice   Serves Four

1 *large onion*
1½ *pounds cauliflower*
   florets
1 *8-ounce can tomato*
   sauce
½ *cup water*
2 *tablespoons chopped*
   parsley
2 *teaspoons ginger*
2 *teaspoons cumin*
1 *teaspoon cardamom*
1 *teaspoon coriander*
1 *teaspoon honey*
½ *teaspoon mustard seed*
½ *teaspoon turmeric*
¼ *teaspoon cayenne*
   pepper
½ *teaspoon salt*

Mix all the spices together. In a saucepan, cook the cauliflower and onion in ¼ cup of water for 5 minutes. Add the tomato sauce, spices and the rest of the water. Cover and simmer for about 20 minutes until the cauliflower is tender. When cooked, sprinkle with parsley. Serve on top of cooked brown rice.

173

Millet with Vegetables   Serves Four

2½ cups water
1 cup peeled potatoes
1 cup chopped carrots
1 cup shredded cabbage
¼ cup chopped onion
¼ cup chopped turnip or
   parsnip
½ cup whole millet
¼ cup chopped parsley
¼ teaspoon salt

Place the vegetables in a large stew pot and add 2½ cups of water plus the millet, parsley and salt. Bring to a boil. Then cover and cook on medium heat for 45 minutes. Should the vegetables appear too thick, add an extra half cup of water and cook for an extra 15 minutes.

174

Rice and Garbanzo Bean Casserole

Serves Four to Six

2 cups cooked garbanzo beans (or one 19-ounce can of chickpeas)

2 small, finely-chopped onions

1 red or green bell pepper, chopped small

1 cup long-grain brown rice

½ cup raisins

¼ cup plain, nonfat yogurt

2 minced cloves of garlic

1 teaspoon cumin

¼ teaspoon cinnamon

¼ teaspoon ginger

¼ teaspoon mace

¼ teaspoon coriander

¼ teaspoon cardamom

¼ teaspoon cloves

¼ teaspoon cayenne pepper

2 cups water

Preheat the oven to 350° while you lightly spray an oven-proof casserole dish with nonfat vegetable spray. In a pan sauté the onions and garlic in two tablespoons of water for two minutes. Then add the pepper to the onions and garlic and simmer gently for ten minutes. Add a small amount of water if needed to prevent burning. Then add the beans, rice, herbs, raisins and the two cups of water. Bring to a simmer and turn into the casserole dish. Cover and place in the oven. Bake for 25 minutes at 350°. Remove and stir in the yogurt with a fork as you simultaneously puff up the rice and beans.

Vegetable, Pea and Barley Stew   Serves Four

1 14-ounce can stewed
  tomatoes
2 carrots
1 cup green beans
1 cup frozen corn
  kernels
½ cup green split peas
1 small onion
1 clove garlic
½ cup whole barley
½ teaspoon celery seed
1½ tablespoon lemon
  juice
  pepper

Mince the onions and garlic cloves. Finely chop the carrots. Cut the green beans into one-inch lengths.

Then, into a pan containing 3 cups of boiling water, place the split peas, barley, onions, garlic, stewed tomatoes and celery seed. Cover and simmer for 15 minutes. Then, add the carrots, and simmer another 15 minutes. Then add the corn and green beans and simmer for a final 15 minutes (45 minutes total simmering). Season with lemon juice and pepper.

Vegetable Stew   Serves Eight

4 cups fresh or canned
  tomatoes
2 large cubed potatoes
2 carrots, sliced
2 zucchini, sliced
2 celery stalks, chopped
1 broccoli head, sliced
2 broccoli stalks, finely
  sliced
2 large onions, sliced
  and chopped
2 tablespoons chopped
  parsley
1 tablespoon paprika
1 tablespoon chili
  powder
1 tablespoon basil
½ teaspoon dry mustard
¼ teaspoon ground
  cumin

In a large stewpot sauté the potatoes, onions, carrots, garlic and celery in a small amount of water for ten minutes. Then add the remaining ingredients. Simmer gently until all vegetables are cooked. Serve with whole grain bread.

Stuffed Zucchini   Serves Four to Six

1 8-ounce can tomato
sauce
4 carrots, finely sliced
2 stalks celery, finely
sliced
²/₃ cup dried lentils
1 medium onion,
chopped
½ green pepper, chopped
2 cups water
4- 6 medium zucchini
(one per serving)
½ cup whole wheat
bread crumbs
2 tablespoons fresh
parsley, chopped
2 cloves minced garlic
1½ teaspoons dill weed
1 bay leaf
½ teaspoon dried
marjoram
½ teaspoon dried
tarragon
¼ teaspoon dried thyme
pepper

Place the water, onion, lentils, carrots, green pepper and bay leaf in a large pan. Simmer gently for about 35 minutes, until the lentils are cooked and most of the water has been absorbed. Remove the bay leaf. Next, parboil the whole zucchini in boiling water for 10-15 minutes until tender. Drain and cool for a few minutes. Preheat the oven to 350°. Spray a medium-sized baking pan with nonfat vegetable spray. Slice each of the zucchini lengthwise in half. Scoop out the zucchini centers and place in a collander to drain

Arrange the zucchini shells in the baking pan and sprinkle with pepper. Stir the zucchini centers into the lentil-vegetable mix. Next, add the tomato paste, the ½ cup of bread crumbs and the garlic, dill, marjoram, thyme, tarragon and some additional pepper. Fill each zucchini half with the lentil mixture. Bake for about 25 minutes.

If any lentil mix is left over, place in a casserole dish and bake at the same time.

178

Broccoli Medley   Serves Four

1 *bunch broccoli florets*

1 *medium onion,*
  chopped

1 *yellow summer*
  squash, sliced

1 *sweet red pepper,*
  chopped

4- 6 *mushrooms, sliced*

½ *cup vegetable stock or*
  water

2 *tablespoons soy sauce*

2 *tablespoons cornstarch*

Stir-fry the vegetables in water for 2-3 minutes. Add the stock or water, cover and cook until tender. Next, blend cornstarch with soy sauce, add to vegetables, and cook till thickened.

179

Pasta and Beans   Serves Four

1 grated carrot
1 rib of celery, chopped
1 large onion, chopped
2 garlic cloves, chopped
1 eight-ounce can
   tomato sauce
1½ teaspoons dried,
   mixed herbs (such as
   basil, oregano,
   marjoram, rosemary
   or savory)
2 cups water or
   vegetable stock
8 ounces wholewheat
   pasta (noodles,
   spaghetti, macaroni
   etc.)
2 cups cooked red or
   kidney beans
   salt and pepper to
   taste

Any kind of whole wheat pasta goes well with this recipe; noodles are fine. Simmer the carrot, celery, onion, garlic cloves, tomato sauce, herbs and water or vegetable stock together for 15 minutes. Then add the pasta and cook for another 15 minutes. Finally, add the two cups of cooked red or kidney beans and stir in.

Squash and Rutabaga   Serves Four

2 lbs winter squash,
  sliced
½ lb rutabaga, sliced
4 garlic cloves, chopped
⅓ cup parsley, chopped
¼ cup whole wheat
  bread crumbs
¼ cup whole wheat flour
  salt and pepper to
  taste

Steam the squash and rutabaga together for 20 minutes, or until tender. Mix together the parsley, garlic, bread crumbs, flour, and salt and pepper and combine with the squash and rutabaga. Then place in a casserole dish and bake at 350° for 30 minutes.

Tamale Bake   Serves Four to Six

1 No.2 can tomatoes
(fresh can be used
instead)
1 No. 12 can whole
kernel corn (fresh or
frozen corn can be
used instead)
2 teaspoons chili powder
¾ cup chopped onion
1 cup soy protein
1 package corn muffin
mix
additional seasoning
to taste

Thoroughly mix all the ingredients except the corn muffin mix in a medium-to-large saucepan. Then, while stirring, heat slowly until the mixture reaches the boiling point. Pour the mixture into a shallow two-quart baking or casserole dish.

Prepare the corn muffin mix according to directions on the package. Cover the corn-to-mato mix in the baking dish with the corn muffin mix. Then bake in a hot oven for 30-40 minutes, until the corn muffin mixture is baked.

You can add more soy protein as needed. Soy protein is available at most health food stores.

CHOLESTEROL CUTTER #9:

HOW TO FIND HEART-FRIENDLY FOODS WHEN EATING OUT

To dine out the low-cholesterol way, choose a restaurant that has a large, well-stocked salad bar. For a few dollars, help yourself to a huge, fresh salad followed by a plate of cooked vegetables, grains and beans, with a dessert of fresh fruit. The only caveat is to watch out for high-fat dressings and sauces. Usually at least one salad dressing is low-fat and sometimes nonfat.

Today, most good restaurants serve at least one low-fat dish, usually baked fish with a choice of nonfried vegetables. Almost any restaurant will prepare a vegetable plate on request. You can ask that all butter, dressing and sauces be omitted.

Other restaurants may feature a large chef's salad as an entree. If you order one, ask that any eggs, cheese, or meat be left out and that any dressing be served on a side dish. You can then use as little of the dressing as possible. If meat, eggs or cheese cannot be omitted, remove them yourself before eating.

Otherwise, the safest bet at any quality restaurant is to order fish, free of oil or butter and, of course, never fried. A standard restaurant portion of fish weighs about six ounces, equal to one day's entire flesh food ration for the Easy-Does-It Plan. Those following the Chol-Tamer Plan can request a doggy bag to take home half their ration.

Most Indian restaurants serve a vegetarian dish with boiled rice and a minimum of fried vegetables. Chinese, Japanese and oriental restaurants also usually serve at least one rice and vegetable dish. Just make sure that neither is fried. Spaghetti, without meat or butter, is an option in most Italian restaurants.

Most Mexican restaurants in the U.S. serve the fat-and-cheese laden cuisine of northern Mexico while low-fat dishes like beans, rice and fresh hearth-baked corn tortillas are considered peasant food. More authentic Mexican restaurants may have baked fish dishes *a la Veracruzana* or some of the nonfried seafood dishes of the Pacific coast. One vegetarian friend of ours always orders a guacamole salad when in a Mexican restaurant. In any case, watch out for frijoles refritos or beans refried in lard.

Regrettably, fat lurks in almost every restaurant. Even natural foods and vegetarian restaurants sometimes sauté vegetables and make liberal use of cheese, oil, butter, and cream. All too many restaurants still deep-fry popular foods. Whether using saturated or unsaturated oils, the oil is kept heated at very high temperatures and is used repeatedly, rendering it extremely dangerous to your health.

You need to watch particularly for fried, deep-fried or sautéed vegetables. When fried, vegetables tend to sop up more fat than even meats. Eggplant, in particular, literally sponges up fat when fried. A single meal of vegetables fried in butter can set back your cholesterol-lowering program by several days. While stir-fried vegetables *are* lower in fat, it's safest to eat only vegetables that are boiled, broiled, steamed or baked.

Fast Food Eateries—Archenemy of Arteries

Provided you watch for high-fat dressings and sauces, cafeterias offer a choice of nonfried vegetable and pasta dishes and baked potatoes and fruit desserts. But all too often, the best thing about fast food chains is the clean bathrooms.

Although some have made a few token concessions, like frying in vegetable oil instead of animal fat, the typical fast food meal still gets 40-50 per cent of calories from fat.

If there is one, the salad bar is the place to head for. Otherwise, despite the reduced-fat milk shakes and the cholesterol-free egg substitutes, it's difficult to walk out of a fast food eaterie without a hefty load of total fat.

Most of us living the low-cholesterol lifestyle soon learn that menu terms like "crisp" or "crispy" are euphemisms for "fried." Among restaurant foods to stay away from are all fried foods, fries and chips, and luncheon meats, burgers, cheeseburgers, hot dogs, frankfurters, sausages and shakes.

Focus instead on chicken and turkey, tuna in water, fish dishes and pasta. If chicken is served with the skin on, simply cut it off and don't eat it. We've often ordered steamed vegetables served dry, with steamed rice and a baked potato with chives. Skip any high-fat dessert or ice cream. Fruit, even canned, is far safer and often tastier.

Many good restaurants today serve breakfast buffet-style with a choice of oatmeal and other cereals, and a variety of fresh fruits. In roadside restaurants, you can still usually order a bowl of oatmeal or grits. We've frequently ordered a bowl of each plus a baked potato—always specifying "without butter or cream." Whole wheat toast spread with preserves instead of butter is reasonably safe.

Having read this far, you are undoubtedly aware that eating a hamburger on a whole wheat bun isn't going to neutralize the saturated fat. But that same kind of hype lies behind the proliferation of bran muffins and cookies listed on breakfast menus.

In reality, many of these baked goodies contain less than five grams of oat or other bran per ounce—not much more than a trace. To digest any worthwhile amount of soluble fiber, you'd have to eat an entire pound of muffins or cookies at a cost of 1,000 calories in fat, sugar and refined carbohydrates.

CHOLESTEROL CUTTER #10:

HOW CARBOHYDRATE LOADING CAN OVERCOME YOUR CRAVING FOR FATTY FOODS

Are you hopelessly addicted to high fat foods like hamburger, fries, ice cream and chocolate? Researchers have discovered that millions of Americans have an uncontrollable craving for these, and other high fat foods, because of their high ratio of fat-to-carbohydrates. The higher the fat content of any food, the easier it is to become addicted to its taste, sensation and texture.

Since infancy, most of us have been programmed to enjoy, and to crave, foods high in fat and low in carbohydrates. Thus the fat-to-carbohydrate ratio of any food determines our degree of addiction.

Fortunately, there's an easy way to thwart and overcome this dangerous craving. It simply consists of making the first course at each meal a complex carbohydrate dish completely free of any fat, oil or butter.

For example, begin dinner with a medium-sized bowl of vegetable soup and whole grain bread, or a bowl of pasta, or a generous vegetable salad. Linger over the first course for 15 minutes or so to give the carbohydrates time to satisfy your hunger craving.

At this point, begin to eat your usual high-fat meal. Most people find that they are feeling so satisfied already that they are unable to eat their customary amount of fat.

If you're unable to spend this long over a meal, eat a high-carbohydrate snack thirty minutes before your next high-fat meal. Try a slice of whole grain bread spread with yogurt cheese and slice a banana or cucumber on it as you eat. Or eat the banana alternately with the bread. Or eat a hollow whole wheat pita bread stuffed with salad vegetables.

Carbohydrate loading is an established nutritional principal for balancing a person's fat-to-carbohydrate ratio. Hundreds of professional nutritionists have used it successfully to help their patients cut their cravings for high-fat foods.

CHOLESTEROL CUTTER #11:

MINI MEALS MAY HELP LOWER CHOLESTEROL

Several anthropologists have speculated that, as gatherers of plant foods, man's early ancestors developed genes that programmed their digestive systems to evolve around frequent nibbling rather than around eating large meals. Supporting this very plausible hypothesis is the discovery that eating large meals triggers the release of copious amounts of insulin which stimulates production of an enzyme that boosts cholesterol production by the liver.

This discovery was confirmed by a small yet careful study authored by David Jenkins, M.D., Ph.D., professor of medicine and nutritional science at the University of Toronto, and reported in the *New England Journal of Medicine* in 1986. In the study, seven men consumed a typical diet (2,700 calories of which 33 per cent was from fat) following a conventional three-meals-a-day routine for 14 days. For the next 14 days, the men consumed the same amount of food in the form of 17 small snacks eaten at one-hour intervals throughout the waking day.

After 14 days on the snack program, their average total cholesterol was 8.5 points lower than on the three-meal routine while their average LDL level had fallen a significant 13.5 per cent. Meanwhile, their average blood insulin level had fallen a dramatic 28.5 per cent.

The study confirmed that by splitting one's normal daily calories into a number of small meals equally spread out through the day, the blood insulin level experiences a significant drop and it takes the total cholesterol and LDL levels down with it.

Besides raising cholesterol, high insulin levels are believed to injure artery walls, laying the foundation for arterial blockage. Eating smaller meals avoids this risk.

Several previous studies made during the 1960s and 1970s observed similar results. One researcher obtained almost equal benefits by dividing up the day's rations into only nine mini meals, equally spaced out throughout the waking hours.

Such a routine would simplify eating mini meals while at work. For example, you could have one snack on rising, one before starting work, one at the mid-morning break, one at lunch time, one at the mid-afternoon break, one on quitting work, and another on arriving home. Cooked meals could be prepared during the evening.

Obviously, sandwiches of whole grain bread spread with yogurt cheese and filled with salad vegetables would make ideal mini meals to eat away from home. So would hollow whole wheat pita bread stuffed with salad vegetables. Or plain fresh fruit.

By contrast, the very worst eating routine is to start the day with no breakfast, to have a Danish or similar nutritional disaster for lunch, and to eat a huge, high-fat, high-protein dinner.

Several earlier studies also found that eating mini-meals

helped to reduce weight and blood pressure and to alleviate some digestive problems. Whatever you can do towards achieving a mini-meal routine is likely to help lower your cholesterol and to benefit your health. Just make sure that your total food consumption does not exceed the amount you would normally eat in your three usual meals.

Caution: if you have any condition which might be adversely affected by following a mini-meal eating program, check with your doctor before adopting this routine.

CHAPTER EIGHT

The Physical Approach

Both exercise and weight loss have a powerfully beneficial effect on cholesterol levels.

A study of 138 men by Paul T. Williams, Ph.D., of Lawrence Berkeley Laboratories, Berkeley, California, found that distance runners have an average HDL level 25–50 percent above normal. Williams and his colleagues concluded that the HDL increase was due primarily to loss of body fat resulting from the effects of both exercise and weight loss. The study also revealed that secretion of the enzyme lipoprotein protase during exercise causes an immediate increase in HDL (the good cholesterol).

EXERCISE—A PROVEN CHOLESTEROL FIGHTER

A tidal wave of medical studies is demonstrating that a brisk daily walk can benefit every part of the body right down to our arteries, cells and cholesterol levels.

For instance, a seven-year study of 540 healthy women aged 42–50 made at the University of Pittsburgh (and reported in *Preventive Medicine,* March 1990) found that women who burned 2,000 or more calories per week in rhythmic exercise had significantly higher levels of HDL, and significantly lower levels of LDL, total cholesterol, triglycerides and blood pressure.

As far back as 1969, researchers like Jan L. Breslow, M.D., of Rockefeller University, New York City, were showing that exercise speeds up clearance of triglycerides from the blood stream.

Then came the large, well controlled Harvard Alumni Study analyzed by Dr. Ralph Paffenbarger of Stanford University which concluded that men who expended 2,000–3,500 calories per week on rhythmic exercise, such as brisk walking, reduced their risk of dying in any one year by 28–40 per cent.

Another eight-year study of 13,000 healthy men and women at the Institute for Aerobics Research, Dallas, reported that the least fit men in the study died eight times more often from heart disease, and four times more often from cancer, than the most fit men. Among women in the study, those who were least fit died nine times more often from heart disease and sixteen times more often from cancer than those who were most fit.

Putting together the results of these, and dozens of similar studies, proves that regular rhythmic exercise bestows clear and unmistakable benefits on every person's lipid profile.

Regular aerobic (rhythmic) exercise is the one best way to raise the level of HDL cholesterol while simultaneously helping to lower the levels of triglycerides and at least a dozen other risk factors that contribute to raising cholesterol.

Exercise Buoys Your Emotions

For instance, regular exercise helps tone up every muscle in the body, including the smooth muscles that surround the coronary arteries. It is these same smooth muscles that keep arteries flexible and dilated. Exercise also increases activity of tissue plasminogen activator, a protein produced by blood vessels that may help to dissolve cholesterol. Exercise also reduces weight and proportion of body fat, excretes coagulants that might otherwise cause a blood clot, boosts self-esteem, and defuses stress, depression and anxiety. A brisk, half-hour walk also releases clouds of endorphin in the brain, creating an exuberant feeling of relaxation and well-being that lasts for hours.

Despite these incredible benefits, the Centers for Disease Control (CDC) report that fewer than eight per cent of adult Americans exercise sufficiently to benefit their health. A large body of scientific evidence exists to show that people who fail to exercise experience a gradual but inexorable decline in all body functions. In sedentary people, the capillaries and small arteries may begin to close down, adversely affecting hormones that regulate everything from blood pressure to cholesterol levels. As the HDL cholesterol level drops, injuries to artery walls multiply while physical deterioration and rapid aging occur throughout the body. Virtually every study has found that an inactive lifestyle increases risk of high cholesterol, hypertension, heart disease, stroke, cancer, diabetes, kidney disease and osteoporosis.

192

CHOLESTEROL CUTTER #12:

WALKING AWAY CHOLESTEROL

When exercise is combined with a low-fat diet, the two factors work synergistically to promote lowering of LDL while maintaining the level of HDL or even raising it. Hence the question is not whether we should take up exercise. It is how much and how often we need to exercise.

The majority of studies are saying that for optimal benefits, we need to burn 2,000 or more calories per week through such brisk exercises as walking, jogging, bicycling, swimming, rowing, cross-country skiing or aerobic dancing. On a daily basis, this translates into walking two and a half miles, bicycling eight miles on a fat-tired bike or ten miles on skinny tires, swimming 900 yards, rowing one and a half miles, or dancing aerobically for 35 minutes daily for seven days a week. Since walking is among the most effective exercises and is almost universally available, we'll focus on this activity. During winter, one can walk indoors in a mall or ride a stationary bicycle.

However, if you are unable to walk, any alternative rhythmic exercise will do. According to the CDC, however, stop-and-go activities like golf, bowling or horseback riding offer virtually no exercise benefit at all. For maximum benefit, we should endeavor to keep moving rhythmically without a break the whole time we're exercising.

The American College of Sports Medicine claims that if you're under 45, a non-smoker, not overweight, apparently healthy and free of any risk factors for heart disease, you should be able to begin a fairly easy but gradually-increasing exercise program without further medical screening.

However, since you'll be seeing a physician for your cho-

193

lesterol test (see Chapter 2), we recommend obtaining medical clearance to exercise during this same office visit. On the other hand, if you're over 45, a smoker, are overweight, take drugs of any kind (especially beta blockers) or have hypertension, diabetes, heart disease, elevated cholesterol or any other diagnosed illness, or are sedentary, you will need medical clearance before beginning to exercise.

Stay Within Your Comfort Parameters

These statements assume you will begin to exercise at a fairly low level of intensity, without over exertion or becoming fatigued, that any increase will be gradual, and that you will always stay within your comfort level and will avoid pushing yourself too hard, at least until you have attained a fairly high level of cardiac fitness.

If at any time while exercising you experience a rapid pulse or a pounding heart; extreme breathlessness, a tightness or pain in the chest, jaw or throat, or down the arm; or nausea, vomiting, dizziness, loss of muscle control or increasing pain in joints or muscles, you should stop immediately. If the symptoms persist, you should see a doctor without delay.

These standard cautions aside, the risk of not exercising is at least a thousand times greater than any risk in beginning a gradually-increasing program of brisk walking. Statistically, the risk of having a heart attack while exercising is approximately one in five million for healthy, middle-aged men and one in 17 million for women. For every person who dies while exercising, 100,000 others die in bed or while eating a high-fat meal.

Not true, however, is the widely-held belief that as long

as you exercise vigorously several times a week, you can safely continue to eat a high-fat diet. While exercise complements a low-fat diet, it will not completely offset the hazards of eating a diet high in saturated fat and cholesterol.

Unfortunately, aerobic exercise does not confer immunity from high cholesterol and heart disease. To become completely safe from heart disease, you must achieve a total cholesterol level of 160 mgs/dl, plus letting go of any other cardiovascular disease risk factors.

Calculating Your Personal Heart Target Rate

For most people, brisk walking means covering 3.75–4.25 m.p.h. with arms swinging while breathing moderately hard and keeping your heart rate within your target range. Here's how to calculate your heart target range:

$$220 - \text{Your Age} = \text{Maximum Heart Rate}$$

Your target heart range is between 60 and 80 per cent of your maximum heart rate. Let's say you're aged 45.

$$220 - 45 = 175$$
$$175 \times .06 = 105$$
$$175 \times .8 = 140$$

Your target heart range is between 105 and 140 beats per minute.

You can take your pulse when walking by briefly pausing for ten seconds while you count the number of beats at the wrist. Or you can feel it at the carotid artery pulse in the throat. Multiply your count by six to obtain the number of beats per minute. For maximum benefit, you should en-

195

deavor to remain in the target heart range for at least 20 minutes during each exercise period.

The Three Stages of Exercise Activity

We recommend starting and progressing in three stages.

•Stage 1: Starting slowly and easily, gradually work up to where you are walking briskly, and staying in your target heart rate for 20 minutes three or more times a week. If it hurts at first, slow down or stop and rest. But don't allow a little obvious muscle soreness to put you off. Feel comfortable with your current speed and distance before increasing. Plan your walking schedule ahead of time, be consistent and give it priority over almost everything else.
•Stage 2: Gradually increase your walk until you are staying in your target heart rate for 25 minutes five times a week.
•Stage 3: Gradually increase your walk until you are staying in your target heart rate for 30 minutes five times a week. Additionally, on two other days each week, forget about your target heart rate while you spend 45–60 minutes enjoying a longer walk that, if possible, includes striding up and down as many hills as possible.

Exercise Guidelines for the Three Cholesterol-Lowering Plans

For those on the Easy-Does-It Plan, we recommend concentrating on Stage 1. For those on the Chol-Tamer Plan, we recommend starting in Stage 1 and progressing to Stage 2 and concentrating on maintaining that level. For those on the Blockbuster Plan, we recommend starting in Stage 1, progressing through Stages 2 and 3, then maintaining Stage 3, or even gradually going beyond it.

Exercising at the Stage 2 level expends more than 1,000 calories per week, enough to influence one's HDL favorably, and to benefit the Whole Person. Exercising at the Stage 3 level expends close to 2,000 calories a week and should substantially benefit the HDL and one's entire body-mind.

Regardless of which cholesterol-lowering plan you are following, you don't have to stay in the corresponding exercise stage. Instead of staying in Stage 1, a person following the Easy-Does-It plan can achieve greater benefit by gradually working up to Stage 2 or 3. And don't hesitate to go beyond Stage 3. Studies show that the more energy you expend up to a maximum of 3,500 calories a week, the greater the benefit. One study also concluded that exercising in a target range between 70 and 80 per cent of the maximum heart rate produced the lowest LDL and the highest HDL.

If time won't permit exercising 5–7 days a week, then you must stay with Stage 1. However, you might think about increasing time spent in the target heart range from 20 minutes to 30 minutes.

Or if staying in the target heart range feels tough, multiply the maximum heart rate by .5 and by .7 instead of by .6 and by .8. Later, you can move back up to the higher multipliers. At all costs, avoid overdoing it. Begin at a comfortable level and stay within your comfort zone. The days of no-pain, no-gain are gone. Never push yourself beyond the point where you can converse or hum a tune without gasping for air.

Wear well-cushioned walking or jogging shoes with adequate arch support and ample space for your toes. Lightweight hiking boots are fine for walking on rough surfaces.

Warm up by beginning to walk at an easy pace and increase gradually to your full walking speed. Likewise, cool down at the end of your walk by walking at a slower pace for the last couple of minutes. This will prevent a sudden drop in blood pressure caused by blood pooling in the legs. Drink a glass of water before and after exercising. Carry only ID and leave all money and valuables at home.

The best foods for energy are also the best foods for lowering cholesterol. For high energy, the muscles prefer complex carbohydrates (plant foods) because the fuel they provide is swiftly available and ready for use. Fat and protein take many hours to digest, and instead of being used to fuel muscles, their calories often end up being stored in fat cells all over the body.

Weight Loss—How to Slim Down and Melt Away Cholesterol

The same high-fat diet and sedentary lifestyle that causes high cholesterol also causes obesity. One of every four adult Americans is 30 per cent or more overweight, and millions of others are overweight by a lesser amount. Being overweight has been directly linked to a high cholesterol level, and to dramatically-increased risk of heart disease, stroke, diabetes and cancer.

Some researchers have reported that for every pound a person is overweight, the liver synthesizes an additional 10 mgs of cholesterol each day. Other studies show that being ten pounds overweight raises total cholesterol by approximately 5–10 mgs/dl., and also causes blood pressure to rise. Being overweight also raises the level of LDL, VLDL and triglycerides while suppressing the level of HDL.

Yet obesity remains pandemic in the U.S., while our society encourages people to eat more and more fattening foods, and to exercise less and less. To lose weight, however, we have only to do exactly the opposite. That means switching to a low-fat diet and exercising more.

To shed surplus pounds we need only adopt the advice given earlier in this book under each Cholesterol Cutter from #2 to #12. As we steadily lower our cholesterol, it is almost inevitable that, if we are overweight, we shall simultaneously begin to lower weight.

So there's no problem about *how* to lose weight.

CHOLESTEROL CUTTER #13:

LOWERING CHOLESTEROL BY LOSING BELLY FAT

What we need to look at is *where* our surplus weight, if any, is located. Having it around the waist can be much more dangerous than carrying extra fat on the buttocks and thighs. Recent studies have shown that the risk is much greater if the surplus weight exists as a paunch, or as a belly spilling out over the belt.

At a recent AHA Convention, Dr. Per Björntorp of Sweden's University of Göteborg reported that having a large belly can increase risk of heart disease, diabetes, stroke, hypertension or premature death by five to ten times.

David S. Freedman, Ph.D., of the CDC has also confirmed that belly fat, generally found in men, is much more dangerous than fat which accumulates in the buttocks and thighs, a condition common in women. Belly fat is easily

199

broken down and transported to the liver where it can elevate insulin and triglycerides levels to dangerous heights. In doing so, it may also raise LDL and total cholesterol levels.

Through eating a diet high in fat, and failing to exercise, men tend to accumulate fat in a spare tire around the waist, making them apple-shaped. An apple-shape frequently indicates a high level of total cholesterol, triglycerides and blood pressure together with an excessively high LDL level and a low level of HDL cholesterol.

Overweight women tend to put on weight around the hips, thighs and buttocks. This makes them pear-shaped. Though women may find this undesirable, being pear-shaped is considerably less risky than being apple-shaped.

Assessing Your Personal Body Fat Hazards

You can estimate your body fat hazard by measuring the circumference of your waist at the navel and dividing it by your girth around the hips and buttocks. Men should measure their hip circumference level with the top of the hip bone, while women should measure their girth at the widest point between hips and buttocks.

The formula looks like this:

$$\frac{\text{waist circumference in inches}}{\text{Hip girth in inches}} = \text{waist-hip ratio}$$

For a woman with a waist of 31 inches and a hip girth of 36 inches, the ratio would be .86. For an out-of-shape man with a waist of 41 inches and a hip girth of 39 inches, the ratio would be 1.1.

The upper acceptable limit for men is considered to be .85 − .9. For women, it is .75 − .8. Higher ratios are considered a possible diagnostic indicator of high lipid levels in the blood stream.

Bald Men May Have Higher Cholesterol

Because men with paunches also tend to be stocky, many also show evidence of male-pattern baldness. According to a study of Neapolitan factory workers by Maurizio Trevisan, M.D., associate professor of preventive medicine at the State University of New York, Buffalo, men with a receding hairline and bare crown tend to have a total cholesterol level that averages 5.9 mgs/dl higher than non-bald men.

Other visible signs that could indicate an above-average total cholesterol include lumps of fat under the eyes, on the Achilles tendon, and on the back of the hands. Move your fingers to reveal the small tendons under the skin on the back of your hands. Visible lumps of fat on these tendons could be an indicator of high cholesterol.

Some physicians regard a white ring or band on the cornea of the eye (a transparent tissue covering the iris and pupil) as a strong indicator of high cholesterol. Naturally, not all people with visible fat have high cholesterol readings. But if you have any of these signs, it would be a good idea to have your cholesterol levels checked fairly soon.

Getting Rid of an Apple-Shaped Abdomen

If you're a man with a waist-to-hip ratio of 1 or more, or a woman with a ratio of .9 or more, you should make a special effort to slim down to your recommended weight and to flatten your tummy. Total fat in the diet is the principal cause of obesity. Since *any* type of fat can cause obesity, it's important to make every effort to cut as much fat from your diet as you can.

If you have *fully* adopted the Chol-Tamer or Blockbuster Plans, you should not need to make any other dietary changes. You should gradually lose weight because these eating plans are low in fat and high in fiber. If you're like most overweight people, regardless of how much high fiber food you eat, you should gradually lose weight. And you'll continue to feel full of energy because the food you are eating consists of high-energy complex carbohydrates.

You should, however, make a special effort to gradually work up to the Stage 3 exercise level described in Cholesterol Cutter #12. Several recent studies have shown that exercising for an extended period of time burns off more fat than a short, intense workout. So as you progress to a higher level of cardiac fitness, consider lengthening your exercise periods so that you go for a longer walk, a longer swim, or a longer bike ride.

A belly spilling out over the waist is known as an abdominal obesity. To flatten the tummy, floor exercises such as sit-ups and leg raises have been traditionally used to strengthen the abdominal muscles. But, these exercises can cause minor back pain and strain in some cases. Instead, today's exercise physiologists recommend doing crunch-ups instead of sit-ups, and leg-lowering instead of leg raising. Both are equally effective at developing the abdominal muscles. But they eliminate just about all risk of injuring the back.

Exercises for Abdominal Obesity

To do crunch-ups, lie flat on your back on a rug on the floor. Knees should be bent at about 90° with feet flat on the floor. Clasp the hands behind the head. Then, keeping the back flat on the floor, raise your head, neck and chest up off the floor and crunch-up as high as you can go. Hold a moment, then lower your head back to the floor. Exhale as you crunch-up and inhale as you lower back down. As you build strength, do 20–30 crunch-ups per session.

To strengthen the abdominal muscles by leg-lowering, lie flat on your back on a rug on the floor. Arms should be close to the sides with palms facing down. Legs remain straight throughout the exercise.

Without straining, raise one leg to an angle of about 40° and hold. Raise the other leg to the same angle so that both legs are together. Then, while breathing steadily, slowly lower both legs back to the floor. Lowering the legs should take about 20 seconds. As you gain strength, you can gradually build up to where it takes 30–40 seconds to lower the legs. By raising only one leg at a time, and by raising only to 40°, you avoid any risk of back injury.

Repeat the exercise as many times as you can without strain or discomfort, up to a maximum of ten times. These two exercises can be done once a day or more often.

If you plan to do these or any other exercises, obtain your doctor's permission at the time you take your cholesterol test. Note that any recommendations to lose weight apply only if your weight is above the recommended weight for your height and build. There is no advantage to losing more weight if your weight is normal.

CHAPTER NINE

The Nutritional Approach

Exciting news from the cutting edge of nutritional research is showing that vitamins and minerals are often important catalysts in a number of biochemical processes that help keep cholesterol in check. Moreover, a group of nutrients called anti-oxidants may have the power to almost completely halt further deposits of artery-blocking cholesterol.

However, popping a handful of supplements is not a substitute for eating plenty of fruits, vegetables and whole grains each day, nor for the other salutory habits described in this book. While consuming nutrients vital to heart health may reinforce the success of other Cholesterol Cutter techniques, they should not be relied on alone to bring about a major reduction in cholesterol.

Thus the nutritional steps in this chapter are intended primarily to boost the effectiveness of the other natural cholesterol-lowering methods described in this book. And since it certainly enhances your overall nutrition, cutting back on caffeine is also described here.

CHOLESTEROL CUTTER #14:

NUTRIENTS THAT MAY HELP LOWER CHOLESTEROL

As insurance against the slight possibility that a high-fiber diet may inhibit absorption of some vitamins or minerals, several nutritionists have suggested taking a daily multi-vitamin-mineral supplement which provides the minimum RDA for each nutrient. Since nutrients interact synergistically, it is best to take a supplement that includes the RDA for the entire range of vitamins and minerals.

Among individual nutrients, niacin (nicotinic acid or Vitamin B-3) is best known for lowering cholesterol. To be effective, however, the dosage must be 75–250 times the RDA. At these huge amounts, niacin becomes a drug and must be taken only under medical supervision. Although it's the least expensive cholesterol-lowering drug, it can be unpleasant to take, compliance is poor, and among possible adverse side effects are hepatitis or liver damage, kidney failure, breathing difficulties, peptic ulcer, gout, headache, itch, rash and persistent nausea. Niacin may be cheap but it's still a high price to pay for the privilege of continuing to eat fat.

Niacin has no effect in small doses and it should never be used if your triglycerides level is over 150 mgs/dl and your HDL is under 40.

Nutrients That Neutralize Free Radicals

Strong indications are emerging from cholesterol research that LDL (the bad cholesterol) must be oxidized by free radicals before it can create artery blockage. (The free radical theory of cholesterol blockage is described in full in Chapter 4 under the heading "How free radicals create cholesterol plaque.")

Briefly, red meat, polyunsaturated vegetable oils and other fats become chemically rancid when exposed to heat, air or digestion. In the process, they release renegade particles called free radicals which, among a long list of other molecular mayhem, oxidize LDL particles in the bloodstream or liver.

Non-oxidized LDL is recognized as "self" or non-threatening by the body's immune system. But oxidized LDL is so changed that our immune system identifies it as "non-self" or foreign and potentially dangerous. To safeguard the body from this possible hazard, the immune system's large scavenger cells (called macrophages), engulf and swallow up all oxidized LDLs.

By a process not yet fully understood, these LDL-bloated macrophages are lured into tiny cracks or injuries in artery walls where they become embedded and protrude out, partially occluding the artery. The destructive activity of free radicals released from fats in the diet is now believed key to the formation of artery blockage.

Meanwhile, strong evidence is also emerging to show that a group of nutrients known as anti-oxidants are able to inhibit—or even to entirely stop—the formation of cholesterol plaque in coronary arteries by their ability to neutralize free radicals.

Since free radicals may also contribute to several types of

cancer as well as to conditions such as cataracts, anti-oxidants may well be the nutrients of the future.

These anti-oxidants are vitamins A (as beta-carotene), C and E and the mineral selenium.

Beta-Carotene—Terror of Free Radicals

Found in yellow-orange fruits and vegetables and in some deep green leafy vegetables, beta-carotene is the chemical parent of Vitamin A. Unlike supplemental Vitamin A, which is harmful in large amounts, it is impossible to overdose on beta-carotene. The body simply draws on this nutrient as it is needed.

Several studies, some reported at the 64th Scientific Session of the AHA in 1992, have confirmed the role of beta-carotene in protecting the body from coronary artery disease. In the Nurses' Health Study, a multi-purpose study of 87,245 women monitored for eight years, a high intake of fruits and vegetables rich in beta-carotene, (or beta-carotene supplements) was associated with a 22 per cent reduction in heart disease risk and a 40 per cent reduction in risk of stroke.

Yet another large-scale study, Harvard Medical School's Physicians' Health Study, which traced 22,000 male physicians over a ten year period, showed that men with a history of cardiac disease, who took a 50 mgs beta-carotene supplement every other day, had half as many deaths from stroke and heart disease as did a control group taking a placebo.

Researchers report that a daily intake of 25 mgs of beta-carotene provides adequate protection. A single carrot supplies 15–20 mgs per day. Other good sources of beta-carotene are yams, canteloupe, broccoli, apricots, pink grapefruit, red peppers, mangoes, peaches, papaya, sweet potatoes, pumpkins, yellow squash, spinach, kale, collards and dark green romaine lettuce. For those unable to eat fruits or vegetables, beta-carotene is also available in supplement form.

Vitamin C—The Free-Radical Destroyer

Lab tests show that Vitamin C is the most effective of the anti-oxidants in blocking LDL oxidation. It appears to entirely halt macrophages from gorging on oxidized LDL. Other tests reveal that a higher dietary intake of Vitamin C is invariably associated with higher levels of HDL.

Among studies to confirm this finding is the prestigious Baltimore Longitudinal Study of 800 men and women aged 20–95. The study authors report that those participants with the highest levels of Vitamin C showed HDL levels approximately five points higher than those in participants with the lowest levels of Vitamin C. Other tests have revealed that heart attack victims, and people with high blood pressure, almost invariably have low serum levels of Vitamin C.

Vitamin C is also essential to activate the enzyme used for converting cholesterol into bile acid in the liver. Thus an adequate intake of Vitamin C can enhance one's ability to transform cholesterol into bile acid. Soluble fiber in the diet then combines with this cholesterol-rich bile acid and excretes it.

Good sources of Vitamin C include broccoli, brussels sprouts, tomatoes, green peppers, canteloupe, papaya, strawberries, kiwi fruit and oranges (including fresh orange juice). If for some reason you are unable to eat several helpings of fruits and vegetables each day, you might consider taking a moderate amount of supplemental Vitamin C.

A Vitamin That Sops Up Free Radicals

Vitamin E, the principal fat-soluble anti-oxidant, functions wherever fat is present in the body. Tests show that men and women with angina have consistently lower levels of Vitamin E in the bloodstream.

In the same Nurses' Health Study mentioned earlier, taking 100 international units of Vitamin E daily in supplement form was associated with a 36 per cent drop in heart disease risk.

According to the World Health Organization, a low blood level of Vitamin E is the single most important risk factor in death from ischemic heart disease (oxygen starvation of heart muscle due to artery blockage). Based on data from 16 European cities reported in the *American Journal of Clinical Nutrition* (vol 53, #1), low Vitamin E levels were linked to blocked coronary arteries in 62 per cent of deaths from ischemic heart disease. The study's authors cited a low level of Vitamin E as a greater heart disease risk than high cholesterol, smoking or high blood pressure.

Additionally, Vitamin E may also reduce the ability of platelets to coagulate and form blood clots, a major cause of heart attack and stroke. A large study of 36,000 men and women in Finland also found that people with high blood levels of Vitamin E had less cancer.

Many Americans who eat a diet high in refined and processed foods may have a deficiency of Vitamin E. Some natural foods like wheat germ, sweet potatoes and kale contain appreciable amounts of Vitamin E but the principal dietary sources are fatty foods like nuts, seeds and vegetable oils. For this reason, supplements may be the preferred source. Two hundred I.U. per day may be sufficient but many people, including some cholesterol researchers, take 400 I.U. daily. It usually takes several weeks of daily supple-

209

mentation to raise the blood level of Vitamin E to an effective level.

Selenium and vitamin E work together as anti-oxidants. Selenium is a mineral present in grains grown in certain areas. To ensure an adequate intake, a daily supplement of 50–100 micrograms should be ample to maintain anti-oxidant benefits.

Some researchers have also suggested that a deficiency of vitamin B-6, combined with a high intake of animal protein, may lead to an excess of the amino acid methionine. Beef often contains significant amounts of methionine. Methionine is a precursor of homocysteine which causes smooth muscle cells to multiply inside artery walls. Eventually, these surplus cells break away and become part of the debris that contributes to the formation of arterial plaque. All indications are that methionine can be metabolized and rendered harmless by a sufficiency of Vitamin B-6 in the diet.

If you continue to eat a diet high in animal protein, especially beef, you may wish to take a multiple B-Vitamin tablet containing vitamin B-6.

Minerals That May Help Lower Cholesterol

According to a study published in the *British Medical Journal* in 1991, participants who took potassium supplements lowered their total cholesterol by an average of 20 per cent in only eight weeks. Their blood pressure levels also dropped significantly. Most advisory agencies recommend an intake of at least 2,000 mgs of potassium daily for adults. When you consider that a total of five servings of fruits and vegetables daily yield an average 3,500 mgs of potassium, it is apparent that the dietary advice in this book provides an abundance of this mineral. Bananas, potatoes, tomatoes, winter squash, spinach, and broccoli are particularly rich in potassium. While supplements were used in the study, most plant-based foods provide such a rich supply of potassium that supplementation is normally unnecessary.

Among minerals, a deficiency of chromium has been associated with elevated cholesterol. Studies suggest that up to 90 per cent of Americans may have some degree of chromium deficiency, usually due to eating refined and processed foods instead of complex carbohydrates.

Chromium works by helping to lower insulin levels which, in turn, aids in lowering cholesterol and triglycerides levels. An adequate level of chromium in the blood stream is also believed to help prevent injury to artery walls.

Since chromium works synergistically with a variety of other nutrients, it should be taken in the form of a full balanced supplement of all essential minerals. Taking a single supplement of chromium is likely to cause a deficiency of some other mineral. The RDA for chromium is 50–200 micrograms daily.

Currently, one of the most popular chromium supplements is chromium polynicotinate, a niacin-bound chromium complex. According to studies by Dr. Martin Urberg of Wayne State University, when chromium and niacin are taken together, the amount of niacin needed to reduce cholesterol is dramatically reduced.

Where, previously, the minimum dosage of niacin needed to lower cholesterol has been 750 mgs., when combined with 200 micrograms of chromium, the same result was achieved with only 100 mgs of niacin. Chromium polynicotinate, a biologically-active component of Glucose Tolerance Factor, is available in most healthfood stores. In supplement form, it comes in a combination of 100 mgs of niacin and 200 micrograms of GTF chromium.

Manufacturers claim that one small tablet daily is all you

need to help lower cholesterol. While this product may eventually prove to be a less harmful replacement for medically-supervised niacin treatment, mention at this time does not imply our endorsement.

A Vitamin Supplement to the Rescue

Since some people have a problem absorbing one or more minerals from food, taking a full, balanced mineral supplement can be a good idea. Indirectly, virtually all minerals play a role in regulating cholesterol while magnesium and calcium are also essential for regulating blood pressure. Thus any mineral supplement should include at least the RDA of chromium, magnesium, calcium, copper and zinc. We suggest not exceeding the RDA of zinc (15 mgs) since larger amounts may suppress the level of HDL.

Magnesium is a key mineral for protecting heart health. When free fatty acids increase in the blood stream due to emotional stress, the magnesium level is reduced. Stress hormones like adrenalin—released during the fight or flight response—deplete the magnesium level even more while simultaneously raising blood pressure. Since magnesium protects artery walls from damage by sudden blood pressure increases, it is obviously important to maintain an adequate level of magnesium in the blood stream.

Coronary artery spasm is a type of angina caused when the smooth muscles clamp down on the coronary arteries and block the flow of blood to the heart. It can be due to stress or to a deficiency of magnesium, or to a combination of both. In some people prone to coronary artery spasm, supplementation with magnesium and calcium has reduced the frequency of this type of angina and, in some cases, has ended it entirely.

The RDA for magnesium is 400 mgs while for calcium 1,000 mgs is considered adequate for cardiovascular health. Since some magnesium and calcium is contained in the diet, it may not be necessary to take the full RDA amount.

While the supplement amounts mentioned in this section are considered totally safe, we recommend checking with your doctor or nutritionist before taking more than the RDA for any vitamin or mineral. If at any time you have any adverse side effects from taking a supplement, cease taking it at once.

Many Americans Are Deficient in Nutrients Vital to Heart Health

Virtually everyone's basic need for vital nutrients could be met by eating the plant-based diets advised in this book. Supplementation would not be required. The U.S. government's 1990 guidelines urge all Americans to eat 3–5 daily servings of vegetables, 2–4 servings of fruit, and 6–11 servings of breads, rice, pasta and grain.

But government statistics show that, in real life, only nine per cent of adults consumes a total of five servings of fruit and vegetables daily. Everyone else consumes less. And five servings is considered the minimum essential for health and adequate nutrition. The plain fact is that most Americans simply don't like vegetables.

If you are still one of those not meeting the guidelines above, supplements could be helpful. But the fact that you may need supplements is also a warning to redouble your efforts to eat more vegetables, fruits and whole grains.

CHOLESTEROL CUTTER #15:

FAREWELL TO COFFEE

Coffee has been accused of causing everything from high cholesterol to heart disease and cancer. So far, most studies have failed to confirm any really hard correlation. One problem is that many heavy coffee drinkers also smoke and eat a high-fat diet. Nonetheless, due to the uncertainty regarding coffee's role in elevating cholesterol, and in intensifying risk of heart disease, many doctors are recommending that patients with elevated total or LDL cholesterol should either reduce caffeine consumption, or stop using it entirely. No doubt exists, that to some extent, caffeine does stress the heart.

The safe upper limit for drinking coffee has been set at two cups per day. This advice refers to filtered coffee, the type most commonly used in the U.S. Recent studies from both Norway and the Netherlands have found a strong link between rising levels of total and LDL cholesterol and the consumption of boiled coffee, the type most popular in northern Europe.

For example, the Norwegian study found that drinking nine or more cups of boiled coffee per day increased LDL levels by an average of 30 mgs/dl., or 14 per cent. When the subjects in the study ceased drinking boiled coffee for ten weeks, their LDL levels fell by an average of 13 per cent.

The Netherlands study, authored by Dr. Dederick E. Grobbee of Erasmus University Medical School, found that people who drank boiled coffee for nine weeks experienced a ten per cent rise in total cholesterol. Boiled coffee, made by pouring boiling water into a pot of ground coffee, is believed similar to percolated coffee used by roughly 20 per cent of U.S. coffee drinkers.

Based on these and several previous studies linking coffee drinking to increased cholesterol levels, some researchers have suggested that caffeine—even that in filtered coffee—may increase the blood concentration of two cholesterol-binding proteins. Another study recently published in the *American Journal of Cardiology* claimed that total cholesterol rises in direct proportion to the number of cups of coffee drunk.

Yet another study at Johns Hopkins University by epidemiologist Andrea La Croix, found that drinking five or more cups of coffee per day could increase risk of heart disease. Still other studies have shown that drinking two large cups of coffee—about 300 mgs of caffeine—may cause a 50 per cent increase in loss of magnesium and a 100 per cent increase in loss of calcium. Both minerals are essential to the health of heart and arteries. The tannic acid in tea and coffee is also believed to reduce absorption of iron from food. Again, coffee drinking has been linked to arrhythmia, a form of heart disease.

Why You Should Not Drink Decaffeinated Coffee

Nor is decaffeinated coffee safer. A recent study at Stanford University found that drinking three to six cups of brewed decaffeinated coffee per day did raise cholesterol. A similar study at Harvard School for Public Health also found that people who drink more than four cups of decaffeinated coffee per day have roughly 60 per cent greater risk of heart disease than those who do not. The health risk in decaffeinated coffee is believed due to chemicals in the Robusta coffee

215

bean used in making decaffeinated coffee. Thus far, tea de-caffeinated by the water process, appears safe.

Even though some of the links between elevated choles-terol and coffee (or decaffeinated coffee) are statistically weak, both Dr. Dean Ornish and the Pritikin Longevity Centers recommend that coffee be avoided entirely.

A typical cup of coffee contains 30–180 mgs of caffeine, with the average being around 100 mgs. Estimating your daily intake is complicated by the fact that while one standard cup holds about five ounces, a large coffee mug may hold six to seven ounces. Again, an average cup of coffee served in the Eastern U.S., is twice as strong as that served in the West.

Pharmacologists consider 260 mgs of caffeine consumed over a short period to be a fairly high dose while an intake of 500 mgs or more per day is a fairly heavy intake. Tea contains less than half the caffeine in coffee but a cup of very black tea can still contain 100 mgs. Lesser amounts of caffeine are commonly found in caffeinated soda drinks, painkillers, chocolate, diet aids and antihistamine.

Guidelines for the Three Cholesterol-Lowering Plans

For those following the Easy-Does-It Plan, we recommend limiting coffee to two five ounce cups daily, or less. For those following the Chol-Tamer Plan, we recommend drinking not more than one five-ounce cup of coffee daily. Those follow-ing the Blockbuster Plan should eliminate all caffeine entirely.

If desired, two cups of medium-strength tea may be substi-tuted for one cup of coffee. All other forms of caffeine should be phased out entirely, as should decaffeinated coffee.

Where coffee is permitted, we suggest using instant coffee. If you do brew filtered coffee, make it only moderately strong, keep it fresh, and limit intake to a maximum of two cups daily. Since a study at the Veterans Affairs Medical Center, Oklahoma City, recently found that drinking coffee prior to exercise can raise blood pressure, we advise not drinking any type of caffeine-containing beverage before exercising.

To handle the caffeine problem in a restaurant, take along your own herb tea bag. Merely order a pot of boiling water and make an infusion using your own herb tea bag.

If you must withdraw from a strong coffee addiction, do so gradually to avoid a headache. For example, if you drink three cups of coffee per day, during the first week of withdrawal substitute one cup of tea for one of the daily cups of coffee. The second week, substitute a second cup of tea for one of the remaining cups of coffee. The third week, replace the remaining cup of coffee with another cup of tea.

Then, over the following three weeks, use the same technique to replace each of your three daily cups of tea with a cup of herb tea. Within 42 days, you will have phased out coffee entirely.

CHAPTER TEN

The Stress Management Approach— How Stress Overload Raises Cholesterol

A high level of chronic stress can be devastating to our coronary arteries and to our cholesterol levels. Both animal experiments and human studies have shown a strong correlation between chronic stress and the formation of cholesterol plaque in the arteries.

It has been well documented that cholesterol is essential in forming stress hormones. In anyone under stress, the liver responds by producing more cholesterol.

Supporting this finding are the results of a study by Ingrid Mattiason, M.D. at the Malmö General Hospital in Malmö,

Sweden. Some 715 shipyard workers were tested for total cholesterol as part of a survey of 40,000 Malmö residents. Several years later, all the shipyard workers were threatened with unemployment. Soon afterwards, the original 715 men were given another cholesterol test. The men threatened with unemployment showed a 45 per cent increase in total cholesterol compared with a similar-sized group of men whose jobs were safe.

At least a dozen similar experiments have each demonstrated that groups of people under stress—such as students facing an exam, or tax accountants during the tax season—collectively experience a significant rise in total cholesterol. Even in people eating a low-fat diet and exercising, stress can raise total cholesterol to a level higher than it would otherwise be.

Identifying the Stress That Raises Cholesterol

Other studies have narrowed down the stress-cholesterol link to where the exact type of stress that raises cholesterol has been identified. The two causes of stress so identified are: hostile Type A behavior with denial of negative emotions; and a feeling of isolation and alienation.

A landmark study by Redford B. Williams Jr., M.D., professor of psychiatry at Duke University Medical Center, Durham, N.C., revealed that it was not the over-achieving or time pressure components of Type A behavior that led to heart disease but a series of components associated with hostility. These toxic emotions, dubbed "free-floating hostility" by Meyer Friedman, discoverer of the Type A personality, include anger, cynical mistrust, and hostility. Dr. Williams concluded that any male with all three of these traits, is five times more likely to die by age 50 than a person with none of these traits.

Similar traits indentified by other researchers have included fear, unforgiveness, being rude and abrasive, manipulating people, feeling vengeful, being condescending to others, feeling resentful and bitter, being self-centered, feeling isolated and alienated, and being mad at the world.

The Petted Rabbit Study

One study that helped identify the health risks of alienation and isolation was the "petted rabbit" study. At the University of Houston, researcher Robert Nerem placed genetically-similar rabbits on a high-cholesterol diet to promote atherosclerosis. After a few weeks, those in the lower cages showed 60 per cent less artery blockage than those in higher cages.

The explanation was that the lab technician, a short person, played with the rabbits in the lower cages during the lunch hour but was unable to reach those higher up. The rabbits in the upper rows were isolated and ignored.

At least a dozen other major studies have validated the fact that cholesterol and heart disease—and, indeed, all chronic diseases—are significantly higher in people who lack a supportive network of family, friends and acquaintances. Loneliness swiftly leads to the sense of alienation and isolation which can raise cholesterol levels and accelerate deposits of cholesterol plaque in artery walls.

Denying the existence of negative emotions is yet another counter-productive trait that can elevate cholesterol levels for a prolonged period. In a study of 114 young men and women, psychologist Raymond Niaura and colleagues at

Miriam Hospital, Providence, R.I., found a dramatic difference in total cholesterol between those who had a low anxiety level and those who repressed anxiety. The low anxiety group showed an average total cholesterol of 160 mgs/dl while those who buried their emotions, but put on a false happy face, had an average total cholesterol of 200 mgs/dl *plus* a higher average blood pressure and heart rate. This group denied their anxiety but their bodies knew better.

Can We Change the Software in Our Biocomputers?

Suppose we have one or more of these cholesterol-raising personality traits. Are they like a genetic trait? Or can we reprogram our aggressive Type A personality into a relaxed and healthier Type B personality configuration?

A study by psychologist Walter Buckalew, Ph.D., of Cumberland University, used exercise to find the answer. Buckalew discovered that after exercising, people with Type-B personalities showed higher levels of HDL and lower levels of LDL than did people with Type A personalities. One reason, he found, was that while exercising, Type A people tend to display their aggressiveness by competing with, or racing against, other exercisers. Another Type A personality trait was to invariably count laps while swimming and to compete against oneself.

But when the exercisers with Type A personalities adopted relaxed Type B behavior patterns during exercise, Dr. Buckalew found that they had far healthier blood fat levels. Conversely, the study showed that Type A people who competed with—or who raced against—others while exercising, derived less benefit from exercising than did people with non-competitive Type B personalities.

221

Dr. Buckalew's experiments may also help explain why some people with high cholesterol do not experience heart attacks: they may have relaxed Type B personalities.

High Cholesterol Is a Whole Person Problem

The obvious conclusion from all this is that while a low-fat diet and exercise are essential to lowering cholesterol, nonetheless high cholesterol is a Whole Person problem. And to solve it requires a Whole Person approach.

Supporting this conclusion is the fact that a number of physicians in the preventive medicine field, including Dr. Dean Ornish, believe that stress works together with a high-fat diet and the sedentary American lifestyle to raise cholesterol levels and to block arteries.

The Dynamics of Stress

Stress arises when we are faced with a life event that we believe threatens our security, prestige, comfort or pleasure. Whenever we perceive an event as threatening or hostile, feelings such as anger, fear or cynicism are aroused. With hair-trigger speed, the brain transforms these destructive feelings into the biochemical and physiological reactions of the fight or flight response, a primitive survival mechanism.

Immediately, the adrenal glands squirt adrenalin and other stress hormones into the blood stream, placing the entire body in a crisis mode with all systems GO. Smooth muscles constrict arteries throughout the body, and especially the coronary arteries, restricting blood flow, raising blood pressure, and increasing the ability of platelets to clot. Each of these responses intensifies risk of a heart attack. And in a person whose coronary arteries are already partially blocked by cholesterol plaque, there is heightened risk of an immediate heart attack or stroke.

This dangerous emergency state continues to exist for as long as we continue to perceive the world as threatening and unfriendly. In fact, millions of Americans who perceive the world as threatening or hostile—or who feel cynical, anxious or fearful—live in a permanent state of emergency with their fight or flight response constantly simmering.

Meanwhile, the liver pours glycogen into the blood stream to tense the muscles and to keep them charged with energy in preparation for the physical act of either fighting or fleeing. Since neither act is usually possible in modern society, we must remain inactive and filled with tension.

This is a true picture of the state in which many people with hostile Type A personality traits actually live their lives. With their fight or flight response constantly at the ready, hypertension becomes chronic, their blood platelets constantly threaten to clump and form a blood clot, and their total and LDL cholesterol levels remain elevated.

Inappropriate Beliefs Trigger Stress Overload

Yet the entire process is set off by the way in which our belief system programs us to perceive the events in our lives. For example, both Smith and Jones are employed on a production line in a local plant. Unexpectedly, the plant is forced to permanently shut down and both Smith and Jones are unemployed.

Smith perceives it as a total disaster. He sees his job loss as permanent and he fears he will lose his home, furniture and car. Jones, by contrast, perceives his job loss as a heaven-sent release from a boring occupation, and as a wonderful opportunity to train for a new career in the computer field.

It wasn't the life event, the job loss, that was stressful. It was Smith's aggressive Type A belief system that programmed him to perceive his job loss in a negative way—in a way that turned on his fight or flight response and kept his entire body-mind in a chronically-stressful emergency state. By contrast, when Jones perceived the same event through his relaxed Type B belief system, he saw it as friendly and as a magnificent opportunity to strike out for a rewarding new career.

Since life is filled with potential conflicts arising out of job, marriage, money or similar life situations, it is hardly surprising that people with Type A personality traits tend to have higher levels of cholesterol and more atherosclerotic blockage of the coronary arteries.

Are You a Type A or Type B?

Few of us have any doubts as to whether we have an aggressive, uptight Type A personality, or whether we are predominently a relaxed Type B person. Invariably, it seems, we can immediately recognize our own personality traits and can do so with greater accuracy than can any psychological test. Having read this far, most of us by now will already have identified ourselves as either an aggressive Type A or an easygoing Type B.

Stress management techniques are tools for overcoming the destructive effects of this kind of stress. There are two types: 1) Coping; and 2) Transformational stress management systems.

- Through stress-coping systems, such as deep muscle re-laxation and biofeedback, we can learn to prevent the destructive effects of current stress by deliberately relaxing the body-mind.

Through transformational systems, we can learn to prevent future stress by reprogramming the belief system so that instead of perceiving a life event as hostile and unfriendly (as did Smith), we can see it as non-threatening and harmless (as did Jones). In other words, we can learn to replace our health-destroying Type A personality traits with health-enhancing Type-B personality traits. We can't change a life event but we *can* change the way we react to it.

CHOLESTEROL CUTTER #16:

DEFUSE STRESS WITH DEEP MUSCLE RELAXATION

Deep muscle relaxation is a coping technique which dissipates stress and buffers it from harming the body. People with aggressive Type A personality traits and high cholesterol levels can almost always benefit from practicing deep muscle relaxation.

That's because the stress they experience creates an uncomfortable level of tension in the body from which they seek relief by smoking, using tranquilizing drugs, or by using food as a tranquilizer. Whenever they feel stressed, millions of Americans automatically head for the refrigerator. For them, foods high in fat or sugar, or both, become a tranquilizer for tension caused by stress.

Relaxation therapists have demonstrated that mind and

body are intimately associated. When the mind is anxious or disturbed, body muscles are tense. Conversely, when body muscles are relaxed, in just a few minutes the mind also becomes calm and relaxed. When the mind is relaxed, muscular tension arising from stress swiftly melts away.

Relaxation therapists have also concluded that most people with aggressive Type A personalities may not have experienced true relaxation in years. During a 1986 study at the Menninger Foundation, researchers Patricia Solbach, Ph.D. and Joseph Sargent, M.D. found that many of their patients were unaware of how it felt to be deeply relaxed.

Millions of Americans live in such a continual state of emergency—with their fight or flight response constantly simmering—that they have not experienced genuine relaxation for as long as they can remember. Not until they receive relaxation training, are they able to appreciate the difference between states of tension and states of relaxation.

Learning to Identify Tension in the Body

To achieve deep relaxation, we must first learn to recognize exactly what relaxation is and how it differs from tension.

To do so, lie down on your back—on a bed, couch or floor rug—with arms extended slightly from the sides.

Raise the left arm about six inches, make a fist and tense the entire lower arm from elbow to fist. Tense as tightly as you can, and hold it.

Become aware of the very uncomfortable feeling in your left arm as you hold it under tension. Hold the tension for only six seconds. Then release and gently lower the arm. Experience how comfortable it feels as your left arm and hand quickly become relaxed.

Without pause, repeat the same tensing routine using the right arm. As you hold the right arm tense, compare how it feels with the now-relaxed left arm. Hold your right arm tightly tensed for six seconds. Then release and gently lower it.

Never again should you have any difficulty recognizing muscular tension.

Place your awareness now on your face, eyes and jaw. If you're a typical Type-A person, chances are your jaw will ache with tension. You can probably also identify the dull ache of tension in the face and around the eyes. Much of this tension arises from anxiety, hostility or cynicism. Much of it also becomes so habitual that the tension remains even after the negative emotions themselves may have disappeared.

To Enter Deep Relaxation Using Muscle Tensing

Choose a quiet room where you will not be disturbed and unplug the phone. Lie on your back on a bed, couch or floor rug, with a comfortable pillow under your head. Then carry out these steps:

1. Frown hard and move the eyes upward. Hold six seconds, and release.
2. Press the back of your head down on the pillow so that your neck and shoulders are raised off the bed or floor. Hold six seconds, and release.
3. Tense the neck and shoulder muscles as tightly as possible. Hold six seconds, and release. Tense the chest muscles as tightly as possible. Hold six seconds, and release.
4. Raise the right arm six inches off the bed or floor and

clench the fist. Tense as tightly as possible from the shoulder down. Hold for six seconds, and release. Repeat with the left arm.

5. Tense the abdomen muscles tightly. Hold six seconds, and release. Tense both buttocks tightly. Hold six seconds, and release.

6. Raise the right leg six inches off the bed or floor, curl the toes and tense the entire leg and foot as tightly as you can. Hold for six seconds, release, and lower the leg. Repeat with the right leg.

7. Take five, slow deep breaths, filling the abdomen and upper chest each time. Resume normal breathing.

Remain relaxed.

Deepening Your Relaxation Level

Place your awareness on the soles of the feet. Silently say to yourself, "My feet feel relaxed. Relaxation is filling my feet. My feet are deeply relaxed. Relaxation is filling my legs. My legs are limp and relaxed. Relaxation is flowing into my thighs. My thighs feel limp and relaxed."

It isn't necessary to use these exact words. But do give yourself essentially these same suggestions. As you mentally release each body part, place your awareness on that area and visualize it as limp and relaxed. For example, you might visualize your thighs filled with fluffy cotton, and as limp and relaxed as a piece of tired, old rope.

Continue to tell yourself, "My buttocks feel limp and relaxed. My buttocks are as relaxed as if they were filled with cotton. My abdomen is limp and relaxed. My neck and shoulders feel limp and relaxed. My arms and hands are limp and relaxed. My whole body feels as limp and relaxed as a rag doll."

If you detect any area of tension, mentally relax it before going on.

Now place the awareness on the face as you say, "My forehead feels smooth and relaxed. My eyes are quiet. My face is soft and relaxed. My tongue is relaxed. My mouth is relaxed. My jaw is slack."

Check carefully for any remaining areas of tension in the eyes, jaws or temples. If you locate any, repeat the suggestions until the tension subsides.

Finally, tell yourself, "My entire mind and body are deeply relaxed. I am in a state of deep relaxation. I am completely at peace and in harmony with the world. I experience only peace, love and joy. I am thoroughly content and completely at ease."

By now, your mind should be wonderfully clear and receptive and you should be awake and aware of everything that is going on. Let go of the past and the future, keep your awareness on the here and now, and continue to savor and enjoy the present moment.

Dilating the Arteries with Biofeedback

You can now use a simple form of biofeedback to dilate the arteries in your hands and arms and in your feet and legs, and, eventually, throughout your body.

Begin by visualizing yourself lying on a sunbaked tropical beach. Picture a few flecks of white cloud dotting the wide, blue sky. "Feel" a gentle breeze caressing the murmuring surf. And "see" half a dozen white sailboats dotting the green-blue sea.

Picture your hands lying on the sunwarmed sands. "Feel" the texture of the warm sand under your fingers and palms. In your mind's eye, visualize the warmth flowing into your fingers and hands. Use your imagination to experience all the sensations that go with this relaxing scene. "Hear" soothing Hawaiian music as the gulls wheel and screech overhead. "Feel" heaviness creeping into your hands and arms.

Center your awareness on your hands and silently repeat these phrases," Warmth is flowing into my hands. My hands feel quite warm. My hands and arms are warm and relaxed. My hands and arms feel heavy and warm. I feel my hands and arms tingling and glowing with warmth. My mind is relaxed and I am calm and serene. My hands and arms are relaxed and warm."

Gaining Mastery Over Your Involuntary Muscles

Feeding these visual and verbal suggestions to the brain saturates both its hemispheres with powerful affirmations that your hands and arms are becoming heavy and warm. Usually, within a few minutes, one or both hands will begin to tingle, a confirmation of blood vessel dilation. Immediately you feel a hint of tingling in one hand, mentally magnify this feeling and transfer it to the other hand.

If at first you experience tingling only in one or two fingers, don't get discouraged. This is a strong confirmation that you have achieved a high state of relaxation and suggestibility, and that your unconscious mind is carrying out your suggestions. The arteries are beginning to dilate in your hands, allowing more blood to flow in to make your hands warmer and heavier, exactly as you suggested.

Endeavor to notice which mental pictures and suggestions

are most effective. Eventually, most people are able to dispense with the beach scene and they are able to directly visualize warm, fresh blood flowing down the arms and into the hands. They "see" their blood vessels dilate and they "feel" their hands becoming heavier and warmer.

Experiment with other hand-warming visualizations. Try picturing your hands immersed in a bowl of hot water. Or "see" yourself stretching out your hands towards a fire of glowing coals. Use whichever scenes and suggestions work best to warm your hands.

Once you can warm your hands and arms, use the same visualizations and suggestions to warm your feet and legs.

It may take a few weeks of daily practice before you can warm your hands and feet, and your arms and legs. But you *should* be able to reach a state of deep relaxation after only half a dozen sessions.

Inner Surgery Without an Operation

By using visual and mental suggestions to warm your hands and feet, you have employed a basic biofeedback technique designed to relax your arteries and to improve your blood flow. With practice, this effect generalizes throughout the entire body, relaxing and dilating blood vessels everywhere, including the coronary arteries.

As you achieve this deep level of relaxation response, important physiological changes occur. The breathing rate slows from an average of 15–22 breaths per minute to only four to eight breaths. The pulse rate slows and the mind becomes still, clear and calm. The fight or flight reponse is completely turned off and all stress and tension have left the body-mind.

You can continue to enjoy this deeply-relaxed state. Or you can repeat some of the 12 Type B beliefs listed in CC #17.

Returning to Normal Consciousness

To return to normal consciousness, open your eyes, move them around, wrinkle and unwrinkle the face, and move each muscle of the body in turn. Then sit up and move around normally. Try to avoid getting up suddenly.

Since muscle tensing requires a brief but strenuous physical effort, anyone suffering from any form of chronic disease, who is under medical treatment, or who, for any other reason should not undertake muscle tensing or mental suggestions or visualization, should consult his or her physician before attempting any of the techniques described under Cholesterol Cutter #16.

If this caveat applies to you, you may still achieve deep relaxation by skipping the physical act of muscle-tensing.

Eliminating Stress Through Meditation

Meditation is another way to achieve mental and physiological healing through deep relaxation. After analyzing 450 studies of meditation made in 23 countries, research psychologist David Orme-Johnson, Ph.D., dean of research at Maharishi International University in Fairfield, Iowa, is convinced that meditation activates pure consciousness, a mental state that heals the mind by transcending conflicts, anxiety and stress then goes on to mobilize the body's physiological healing resources.

Using statistics based on health insurance claims, Dr. Orme-Johnson reports that meditators use doctors and hospitals only half as often as the general public while their rate of cardiovascular disease is many times lower than that of the average American.

Although Orme-Johnson's research was done on transcendental meditation, also known as TM, which was brought to this country by Maharishi Mahesh Yogi in the late 1950s, there appears to be almost no difference between TM and the classic raja yoga form of meditation which has been practiced in India for almost 4,000 years.

Other findings from Dr. Orme-Johnson's studies show that TM relaxes the body and calms the mind while slowing the rate of brainwaves, heartbeat and breathing. Once this state is achieved, TM reduces stress and anxiety levels two to four times as effectively as any other relaxation technique. When practiced daily, it also stimulates a neuro-physical healing of the entire body.

Although no single study appears to have linked meditation with a reduction in total cholesterol, every indication is that a significant drop in total cholesterol must inevitably be associated with the documented decrease in heart disease risk demonstrated by long term meditators.

Meditation is easy to practice. First, select a quiet place where you will not be disturbed. Then sit upright in a chair with your legs uncrossed and both feet on the floor, and with the hands placed loosely on the knees. Alternatively, you can sit cross-legged on a pillow on the floor or ground with your hands on your knees. In either case, sit upright and keep the spine as straight as possible.

Breathe slowly and deeply, filling the abdomen at the start of each inhalation and continuing to fill the lungs to the top of the chest. Then exhale slowly in the opposite sequence, releasing air from the top of the lungs first and the abdomen last. Maintain this deep, relaxed rate of breathing.

Now place the awareness on the breath. "Watch" the

breath, that is, be aware of it as air flows in through your nostrils and as you exhale this same air through the nose or mouth. Concentrate on watching the breath.

Should a distracting thought occur, as it undoubtedly will, witness that thought. Watch the thought without becoming involved in it. Keep your "self" separate from the thought. Usually, the thought will disappear within a few seconds. Otherwise, slide the intruding thought off your inner video screen and return to watching your breath.

Within a short time, your entire metabolism will slow. Tension will drop away from the shoulders, neck and face. And you will experience a wonderful feeling of calm and peace.

Another way to meditate is to silently repeat a word or mantra while keeping your awareness on it. The word or words you use may have a spiritual association such as "hail Mary" or "shalom" or you may repeat the universal yogic sound of "Om." For best results, silently repeat the chosen word to yourself as you watch your breath during inhalation and repeat the mantra again while you watch your exhalation.

Whenever you find your mind thinking a distracting thought or making a mental picture, watch the thought or image until it disappears. If it persists, slide it out of your mind and resume watching your breath and repeating the mantra.

Be careful not to force anything. Don't strive for results. Just watch your breath and/or repeat the mantra. Slowly, imperceptibly, you will find that your mind is freeing itself of anxiety and stress while your body feels rejuvenated and charged with new energy.

For a deeper experience, perform the deep muscle tensing and relaxation routine prior to sitting upright and commencing to meditate.

You may also be interested in joining a meditation group. Among yoga organizations with branches or chapters around the country are Siddha Yoga, Integral Yoga, Kripalu Yoga and Transcendental Meditation. Most branches offer a weekly class which includes breathing, chanting and meditation. Also don't overlook the many classes in various forms of stress management and yoga offered by park and recreation departments, senior centers, community colleges, hospitals, adult education departments and state universities. Such classes not only teach how to lower stress, but they may also bring you into contact with other people who may share your interests.

CHOLESTEROL CUTTER #17:

HOW TO TRANSFORM AN AGGRESSIVE TYPE A PERSONALITY INTO A RELAXED TYPE B.

Stress arises from viewing a life event through a filter of negative beliefs. Relaxation arises from viewing a life event through a filter of positive beliefs.

An axiom of modern psychology is that we can change our personality by changing our belief system. People with aggressive Type A personalities still view the world through a filter of outdated conditioned beliefs that they acquired in early childhood, picked up from parents, teachers, or while in the armed forces. These beliefs may have been appropriate at the time. But they are inappropriate to our lives today. In many cases, they are creating a high level of stress that is destroying our health.

Modern psychology is also rapidly recognizing that only

235

two basic emotions exist: love and fear. The distinguishing feature of an aggressive Type A personality is that it is programmed by a fear-based belief system. Conversely, a person with a relaxed Type-B personality views life through a love-based belief system.

Negative Emotions That Elevate Cholesterol

Upon perceiving a potentially stressful life event, a person with an aggressive Type A personality is very likely to experience such fear-based emotions as anger, hostility, cynicism, anxiety, bitterness, guilt, resentment, frustration, envy, dissatisfaction, hopelessness, helplessness and depression. Experiencing these destructive emotions over a prolonged period may elevate LDL cholesterol, suppress HDL and intensify risk of heart disease and cancer.

Upon perceiving the same life event, a relaxed Type B person is likely to experience feelings of joy, love, peace, generosity, forgiveness, compassion and contentment. Experiencing these health-enhancing emotions over a prolonged period tends to lower LDL cholesterol, raise HDL and may significantly reduce risk of heart attack and cancer.

It may sound simplistic. But an extensive body of compelling evidence offers strong confirmation that we can transform our personality configuration simply by adopting the same love-based beliefs that most people with a Type B personality hold.

In the process, these beliefs will override and replace the old worn-out conditioned beliefs that are ruining our life and health.

All we need do, actually, is to:

1. *Be aware* that it is our fear-based Type A beliefs that

are causing our stress (and in the process, helping to keep our total cholesterol high).

2. *Be aware* that by replacing our aggressive Type A belief system with a Type B belief system, we can cease creating further stress. Instead, we can enjoy feeling good all of the time by living in a constantly relaxed state.

3. Knowing this, all we need do to end stress entirely is *to adopt the following beliefs.*

Type B Beliefs That Can Liberate Us From Stress

1. I know there is nothing to fear. I can help my total cholesterol level to fall as I let go of fear and replace it with unconditional love.

2. I do and acquire only things that will maintain and deepen my inner peace. I cease craving superficial excitement and stimulation. I realise that lasting happiness comes only from contentment and not from things that I do, eat, drink or buy. I am deeply aware that I cannot achieve lasting happiness from eating high-fat foods that send my cholesterol level soaring.

When I am content and at ease, my body and mind are calm and relaxed. My LDL cholesterol level falls and my HDL cholesterol level rises.

3. My birthright is perfect health and a low level of total cholesterol. Perfect health is my normal, natural state.

4. I am content to be wherever I am here and now. I always have everything I need to enjoy the present moment, therefore my needs and wants are few.

5. I think in terms of cooperation rather than competition. I no longer want to race against others during non-competitive exercise and I no longer plan to count laps while swim-

237

ming. Instead, I plan to exercise for a certain length of time at a brisk yet relaxed pace and to enjoy every moment of it.

Knowing that I will derive greater health benefits by holding this belief, I extend it to every aspect of my life. Instead of competing, I will enjoy every moment of every day regardless where I am, how I'm feeling, whom I'm with, or what I'm doing.

6. I view each seeming problem as a challenge, and as a fresh opportunity to grow, to progress, and to learn, and not as a fight against the clock or against another person or another corporation.

7. I forgive and release forever anyone I have not forgiven—including myself. I forgive everyone, everything and every circumstance, totally and right now.

8. Whether in thought, word or deed, I cease to judge, condemn, criticize or attack another person. I see only the best in everyone, including and most especially myself.

9. I have totally ceased to worry about the future. All my fears about the future exist only in my imagination. I am a powerful person and I am completely capable of handling whatever the future may bring. Besides, when it arrives, the future will have become the present.

I also totally let go of the past and with it, all guilt and resentment.

10. I am always optimistic, hopeful, cheerful and positive. I expect good things to happen to me today, tomorrow and throughout life.

11. I love everyone unconditionally, including and most especially myself. I accept everyone the way they are without requiring them to change.

12. I experience only abundance, and I am willing to share my abundance with others. For I realise that giving and receiving are the same. Whatever I give or lose, I will

receive back several times over. (Naturally, this does not apply to gambling or betting nor to "loaning" money to financially-irresponsible people, including members of your own family).

Reprogramming Your Personality

Read through and absorb these 12 affirmations once each morning and evening. During the day, before you make any decision to act, ask yourself if your choice is in keeping with the spirit of these 12 love-based beliefs.

If your job forces you to make choices that are obviously inappropriate, simple accept them for now. Just witness them without reacting emotionally.

You can control your emotions by controlling your thoughts. Just as each thought that enters our mind is determined by the context of the beliefs that we hold, so every feeling we experience arises out of the context of a preceding thought.

Every negative feeling is preceded by a negative thought that arises from holding negative beliefs. Likewise, every positive emotion is preceded by a positive thought that arises from holding one or more positive beliefs.

Although it's difficult to change a negative emotion once it has taken hold, it is extremely easy to slide a negative thought out of mind before it has time to trigger a negative emotion.

By way of example, think about and make mental pictures or images of a friend or neighbor who has a more exciting spouse, a more expensive car, a larger house, or a more prestigious job.

Be warned, though! If you're a Type-A person, you've

239

probably set yourself up for strong feelings of envy and possible resentment. Within a few minutes, these negative feelings can set off low-level stress mechanisms and you will begin to feel tense, uncomfortable and upset.

Obviously, it is difficult to change this stressful feeling once it has begun. Yet it would have been extremely easy to have slid the thought about your friend or neighbor out of your mind the moment it appeared.

How to Feel Any Way You Want to Feel

A thought is identical to a mental picture. To prove how easy it is to change your thoughts, close your eyes and visualize a snow-capped mountain peak. Now slide the mountain off your inner video screen and picture a red rose. Now slide the rose off and replace it with a picture of a dog.

If you were able to visualize these three images successfully, it's proof that you have the ability to control your thoughts. Whenever a negative thought appears in the future, merely slide it out of your mind and replace it with a picture of a tropical beach scene, or a beautiful mountain range or garden, or whatever else turns on calm and peaceful feelings.

At first, the negative thought may reappear. You may have to slide it out of your mind several times. But usually, after half a dozen attempts, your mind gets the message that this thought is unwelcome. By watching our thoughts and reprogramming them, we can actually feel any way we want to feel at any time. And for as long as we continue to hold only positive beliefs and thoughts, we can remain in a delightful state of relaxation for as long as we continue to hold a positive mindset.

We need have no downers or rough days or bad moments and we can continue to enjoy every moment of every day.

"But," you are probably saying, "I couldn't possibly live like that. I need to get mad occasionally so that I can appreciate the calm periods in between. And how can I feel happy unless I have blue periods to contrast them with? Besides, that sounds like being a zombie!"

If this, or something like it, comes into your mind, it could be one of the primary causes of stress in your life. And if you believe that getting rid of this stress would turn you into a zombie, consider this.

We all know what is meant by pressing a person's buttons. In virtually every Type A person, when you say or do something to press their emotional button A, tape X will begin to play. Press their emotional Button B, and tape Y will begin to play. Regardless of how often you set off these buttons, in a Type-A person, the same tape will play over and over enedlessly.

So who is really the zombie? A Type A person? Or a Type B who is free of all the buttons and tapes, and who has the freedom to choose his or her response to any potentially stressful situation?

In real life, the only time we need to experience a fear-based emotion is when we are actually threatened by physical danger. Other "reasons" are often excuses by those who prefer the stimulation of strong feelings to the apparently unexciting alternative of experiencing constant joy, peace and calm.

Psychological Dimensions of Scarcity or Deprivation

As you adopt a Type B mindset, you will no longer operate from a feeling that you don't have enough of something, or that there's not enough to go around, or that what you have is inadequate. Toxic Type A emotions commonly arise out

241

of thinking like this: "If only I had————————I'd be happy and people would love me. If only I had a new car, more money, or a master's degree, I'd be happy and successful."

Expressing feelings like these invariably identifies a person as coming from a fear-based position of scarcity. As a result, we become concerned only with getting. This translates into *getting* more security; *getting* more sex, food and stimulation; or *getting* more power, fame, prestige, possessions, recognition or achievement.

If you recognize scarcity in your own personality, this almost confirms that you hold inappropriate Type-A personality traits. Like all fear-based beliefs, once recognized, scarcity can easily be replaced by adopting the 12 Type B beliefs above.

When we get down to basics, a great deal of our high cholesterol epidemic is due to the stress of chasing the dollar. Millions of Americans *do* manage to achieve financial success. Yet all too often, it keeps them so occupied and busy that they have little time left to enjoy living.

If you have time to enjoy watching a sunset, to experience a peaceful stroll beside a river, to go for a walk or a bicycle ride, or to enjoy your family, you probably have greater abundance than many people who have more money, prestige and possessions, but who have no time left to enjoy them.

And statistics show that people who come from a position of scarcity or lack—typically people with aggressive Type-A personalities—are likely to have a total cholesterol level significantly higher than yours.

CHOLESTEROL CUTTER #18:

HEALING ALIENATION AND ISOLATION

Several prominent researchers in the field of preventive medicine have concluded that social isolation and alienation are among the principal causes of stress, elevated cholesterol and heart disease.

For example, when James Goodwin, M.D. and his colleagues at the University of New Mexico, studied 256 healthy elderly adults, they found that those with the best social support systems tended to have the lowest total cholesterol levels.

When another large epidemiological study of 7,000 residents of Alameda County, California, was analyzed by Lisa F. Berkman, Ph.D., of Yale University and S. Leonard Symes, Ph.D., of the University of California, Berkeley, the researchers confirmed that the more social ties people have, the longer they live and the healthier they are.

It was found that those in the study who were unmarried, had few friends and relatives, and who spurned social and community contacts, had a death rate twice that of those who had the most social contacts. By contrast, those with close intimate relationships, especially marriage, experienced less stress, and fewer diseases of all types, and the lowest mortality rates.

Observations show that people with high total cholesterol, or coronary artery disease, often report feeling alienated and isolated, as well as hostile and cynical. As a result, some psychologists have concluded that, as they grow older, many Americans tend to erect emotional walls to defend and to isolate themselves from others.

243

The result is that millions of Americans have become chronically isolated. They have built an emotional wall that keeps others out of their lives. They have set themselves off and apart from the rest of the world.

Loneliness Kills, Relationships Heal

Solid psychological research has shown that isolation and lack of social relationships can increase stress, raise total cholesterol, and intensify the risk of heart disease. Numerous animal studies, including the "petted rabbit" study mentioned earlier, have demonstrated that isolating oneself from others can shorten life and raise total cholesterol.

Several researchers, including Dr. Dean Ornish, have warned of the hazard of being psychologically isolated and alienated from others. For example, a recent study by Dr. William Ruberman reported in the *New England Journal of Medicine*, and based on interviews with 2,320 male survivors of heart attack, showed that those who were socially isolated and had a high degree of life stress had a risk of death from heart disease and other causes four times greater than did participants in the study who had low levels of stress and isolation.

Thus it is particularly important for single people, and those divorced or widowed, to avoid isolation and to begin to experience a feeling of one-ness with people, nature and every living thing.

Anyone who feels isolated or alienated should start by looking for similarities with others, not differences. Deliberately cultivate a wide network of friends, family, contacts and acquaintances. At all costs, avoid social isolation.

Sign up for volunteer work that brings you into close contact with others; join classes, clubs, singles groups, churches and social organizations of every kind. As you meet new people, open up and reveal your true self. Reveal what is really going on in your life. You'll find it a genuine healing experience to share your problems and to increase your intimacy and communication with others.

Each morning, repeat this affirmation: "I am one with every living thing. I never see myself as separate from others."

If you live in a very small town or remote suburb, it may pay to move to a larger center which has more singles activity.

We Can Choose to Be Heart Healthy

The greatest medical discoveries of recent times are not CAT scans, atherectomies or other hi-tech achievements but the discovery that each of us can choose to take complete charge of our health. Tremendous new breakthroughs in cholesterol research have taught us how to lower our cholesterol to the point where heart disease can scarcely exist.

The validity of the Cholesterol Cutter techniques in this book has never been questioned. Millions of Americans are already living longer, healthier and more productive lives through having made our Cholesterol Cutters a permanent part of their lifestyles.

Yet millions of Americans continue to ignore this health advice while other millions erroneously believe they have genetic tendencies that make them heart-disease prone. As their parents, siblings, uncles and aunts are all afflicted with stroke or heart disease by their 60th birthdays, they assume that everyone in the family has inherited familial cholesterolemia and that, regardless of what they do, they too are destined to die prematurely of artery blockage.

While cholesterolemia does run in families, a far more

245

likely explanation is that every member of the family grew up eating the same high-fat diet and learning the same poor health habits from their parents.

Another recent study reveals that short people have greater risk of heart disease than tall people. An outcome of the large Physicians' Health Study, the results were released in November 1991 at the annual scientific meeting of the AHA. The study showed that men under five feet seven inches have 70 per cent more heart disease than those over six feet one. The explanation appears to be that short people have a genetically higher risk because their blood vessels are smaller and narrower and, thus, more easily blocked.

But even if you're only five feet tall and have a family history of heart disease, the fact is that you can still largely offset these risks by concentrating on factors over which you do have control. What we eat, the extent to which we exercise and the way we manage stress are all cholesterol-lowering factors under our direct personal control. By presenting eighteen natural ways through which almost everyone could lower their cholesterol, this book describes the best choices you can make to keep your own personal cholesterol permanently low, and your life healthy and long.

GLOSSARY

Angina. Also called angina pectoris. Chest pain caused when arterial blood flow to the heart is reduced, either by cholesterol blockage or by spasm (constriction) of the coronary artery muscle.

Angioplasty. A surgical procedure to dilate (widen) narrowed coronary arteries by threading a balloon-tipped catheter into the narrowed artery segment. By inflating the balloon, the artery is widened.

Antioxidants. Consisting primarily of Vitamins C and E, beta-carotene, and selenium, and found mainly in plant foods, antioxidants are molecules capable of neutralizing free radicals.

Arachidonic acid. A fatty acid, commonly found in feedlot-raised beef, that may increase risk of a blood clot, heart attack or stroke.

Arrhythmia (or dysrhythmia). An abnormal heart rhythm.

Arteriography. A test in which an X-ray opaque dye is injected into the bloodstream. X-ray pictures can then reveal artery blockage.

Arterioles. Small, muscular branches of arteries. When they contract, blood pressure rises.

Arteriosclerosis. Hardening of the arteries due to cholesterol plaque, or similar conditions, that cause artery walls to thicken and lose elasticity.

Atherectomy. Reaming out a blocked artery with a catheter-tip high-speed cutting drill.

Atheromatous plaque. A lesion protruding into a coronary artery formed of cholesterol, triglycerides, collagen, dead cells and other debris.

Atherosclerosis. A form of arteriosclerosis in which deposits of fat or cholesterol in the inner layer of artery walls causes the artery to narrow.

Artery. A blood vessel with thick but flexible walls that carries blood from the heart to all parts of the body.

Biofeedback. A relaxation technique that dilates arteries, improves blood flow and defuses anxiety.

Blood clot. A jelly-like mass of coagulated blood platelets which seals an injury to prevent blood loss. Blood clots can also clog an artery partly occluded by cholesterol deposits or by artery spasm.

Blood pressure. The pressure in the arteries exerted by the heart in pumping blood.

Capillaries. Microscopically small blood vessels between arteries and veins that distribute oxygenated blood to body cells.

Cardiovascular system. The body's circulatory system consisting of heart and blood vessels.

Carotid arteries. The two principal neck arteries through which flows the blood supply to the brain.

Carotid endarterectomy. Opening up blocked carotid arteries to improve blood flow to the brain and prevent stroke.

Cholesterol. A fat-like substance found only in the tissue of animals, fish and birds, and in egg yolks and dairy products.

Cholesterol baseline. A person's cholesterol baseline is determined by the level of LDL receptors in the liver and is genetically coded. It is the lowest level to which total cholesterol can be expected to drop.

Cholymicrons. The largest type of lipoprotein, cholymicrons have a life of only ten hours and are not included in blood tests for cholesterol.

Complex carbohydrates. Any plant food still in the same whole, unprocessed and unrefined state in which it grows in nature. Whole grain flours and oatmeal are included in this category. Complex carbohydrates are the only foods to contain any appreciable fiber.

Coronary arteries. Two arteries branching off from the aorta that carry oxygenated blood down over the top of the heart where they branch and provide blood to the heart muscle.

Coronary artery disease. Narrowing of the coronary arteries causing reduction of blood flow to the heart.

Coronary artery spasm. Constriction of a coronary artery by muscle spasm, narrowing the artery and reducing blood flow to the heart and causing angina pain.

Coronary bypass surgery. An operation performed to improve blood supply to the heart muscle when narrowed coronary arteries reduce blood flow to the heart.

Coronary heart disease. Conditions created by atherosclerotic narrowing of the coronary arteries which can lead to angina pain or heart attack.

Coronary occlusion. An obstruction in one of the coronary arteries that reduces blood flow to the heart muscle.

Cruciferous vegetables. A health-enhancing family of vegetables that includes broccoli, brussels sprouts and cauliflower.

Docosahexaenoic acid (DHA). See Omega-3 fatty acids.

Deep muscle relaxation. A coping technique based on tensing and releasing muscles that buffers the body from the harmful effects of stress, tension and a Type A personality.

Diabetes. Also called diabetes mellitus. A disease in which the body fails to produce, or to properly use, insulin. Type I (junior-onset) diabetes is inherited while Type II (adult-onset) diabetes is often caused by a high-fat diet, obesity and sedentary living.

DNA (Deoxyribonucleic acid). A long, threadlike spiral helix consisting of two chains of sugar phosphates and hydrogen molecules which forms the nucleus of a cell. In human cells, DNA carries the coding for all genes and all genetic traits and qualities.

Eicosapentaenoic acid (EPA). See Omega-3 fatty acids.

Electrocardiogram (EKG or ECG). A graphic recording of electrical impulses produced by the heart.

Endorphin. Neurotransmitters produced in the brain in response to rhythmic exercise that block pain receptors and create an exuberant feeling of wellbeing that lasts for hours.

Endothelium. The smooth, inner lining of the heart and blood vessels and other body structures.

Familial hypercholesterolemia. A genetic shortage of LDL receptors in the liver and tissues. Unable to find enough receptors to bind to, surplus LDL molecules crowd into the bloodstream, driving up the LDL count.

Free radical. A highly reactive and unstable molecular fragment that has an unpaired electron. Free radicals are capable of damaging cells, DNA and artery walls and, in the process, of causing coronary artery disease and cancer. Free radicals can occur only in fats and oils and in animal foods, especially meat.

Heart attack. Death of, or damage to, the heart muscle caused by an insufficiency of oxygenated blood.

Heart target range. To calculate your personal heart target zone, subtract your age from 220 and multiply the result by .6 and by .8. For maximum fitness benefit your pulse should remain within this range while exercising aerobically for at least twenty minutes on three or more occasions each week. Caution: read Chapter 8 in full before beginning any exercise program.

Heredity. The genetic transmission of a trait or quality from parent to offspring.

High blood pressure. A chronic increase in blood pressure above the normal range.

High-fat diet. Any diet in which 35–40 per cent or more of calories are derived from fat

Hypertension. Identical to High Blood Pressure.

Insoluble fiber. By absorbing water in the intestines, insoluble fiber creates large, soft stools that are associated with significantly lower rates of constipation, diverticulosis, hemorrhoids and colon cancer. It is found in wheat, brown rice and other whole grains, lentils, beans and many fruits and vegetables.

Intermittent claudication. Also called peripheral vascular disease. Intense pain in one or both legs caused by arterial blockage. The pain can be relieved by resting but returns again upon exertion.

Ischemia. Reduction in blood flow to an organ commonly due to obstruction or constriction in an artery.

Ischemic heart disease. Same as coronary artery disease or coronary heart disease.

Lipid. A fatty substance that is insoluble in blood.

Lipoprotein. A lipid enclosed in a protein bubble to make it soluble in blood.

Lipoprotein analysis. Also called a cardiovascular risk profile, heart disease risk profile or coronary risk profile. A blood test that gives a printout of the value of each of the three lipoprotein factors that comprise the total cholesterol level.

Low-density lipoprotein (LDL). The "bad" cholesterol, the principal carrier of harmful cholesterol in the bloodstream.

Low-Fat Diet. Any diet in which ten per cent of calories or less are derived from fat.

Meditation. A method of achieving mental and physiological healing through deep relaxation of body and mind.

Moderate-Fat Diet. Any diet in which twenty per cent or less of calories are derived from fat.

Monounsaturated fat. A type of fat found principally in olive, canola and peanut oil. Although the least harmful of all oils, monounsaturated oils are still 100 per cent fat.

Mortality. The total number of deaths from a specific disease in a population during one year.

Myocardial infarction. See heart attack.

Nitroglycerin. A drug which dilates blood vessels and is frequently used to treat angina.

Occluded artery. An artery in which blood flow has been impeded by a blockage.

Omega-3 fatty acids. A blood-thinning fatty acid found in fatty fish and certain vegetables and vegetable oils.

Palmitic acid. A long-chain fatty acid known to be a powerful promoter of high cholesterol.

Partially-hydrogenated vegetable oils. Oils produced by a manufacturing process which gives a polyunsaturated fat more of the characteristics of a saturated fat. Although widely used in processed foods, these oils are not recommended for heart-healthy eating.

Peripheral vascular disease. See Intermittent claudication.

Plaque. Also known as atheroma, plaque is a deposit of fat and debris in the inner lining of an artery wall.

Platelets. Tiny elements in the bloodstream which can become sticky and lead to blood clots.

Polyunsaturated fats. Liquid vegetable oils such as corn, safflower, soybean and sunflower oil. These oils have been found to lower HDL along with LDL, to foster free radical activity and to be linked to immunosuppression.

Protein. Consisting of amino acids, proteins are the building blocks of the body. An ample protein supply is available from a variety of whole grains, beans and other plant foods. It is not necessary to eat animal protein.

Receptors. Proteins on the surface of liver and tissue cells that bind with lipoprotein molecules. Cells in need of cholesterol grow more LDL receptors while those with a surplus of cholesterol grow more HDL receptors.

Risk factor prediction kit. A software program used by physicians to evaluate risk of heart disease based on eight lifestyle factors.

Saturated fats. A type of fat, solid at room temperature, found in foods of animal origin and in tropical oils and, to a lesser extent, in some fatty plant foods. Saturated fats are the most potent producers of cholesterol in humans.

Simple (refined) carbohydrates. Refined grains, sugar or rice, especially white flour, white sugar and white rice. In the refining process, much of their nutrient and fiber value is destroyed. Alcohol and most sweeteners are also refined carbohydrates.

Soluble fiber. A water-soluble fiber found in oats, rice, corn, beans and other vegetables and fruits that lowers cholesterol by binding with cholesterol-rich bile acids in the intestines and excreting them.

253

Stress. A person's physical or mental tension resulting from his or her response to physical, emotional or chemical factors. Emotional stress can raise cholesterol levels.

Stroke. Also called apoplexy or cerebrovascular accident. A sudden and severe attack caused by an insufficient supply of oxygenated blood to the brain. A hemorrhagic stroke is caused by a bleeding blood vessel or burst aneurysm in the brain while a less fatal type of stroke is caused by a blood clot.

Thrombosis. The existence of a blood clot inside a blood vessel.

Total cholesterol. The sum of the value of each of the three lipoprotein factors in the bloodstream (namely HDL, LDL and VLDL).

Triglycerides. A fat derived from food or that is synthesized in the body from other energy sources, principally carbohydrates.

Type A personality. Considered stressful and hazardous to the health of heart and arteries, a Type A personality is frequently associated with fear, anger, hostility, cynicism and resentment.

Type B personality. A relaxed, heart-healthy type of personality that causes a person to perceive the world as friendly and non-threatening.

Vein. A blood vessel that carries blood from body cells back to the heart and lungs.

Very low density lipoproteins (VLDLs). Another "bad" type of cholesterol. Besides transporting about ten per cent of the body's cholesterol through the bloodstream, VLDLs also carry virtually all triglycerides.

BIBLIOGRAPHY

For Further Reading

Ackart, Robert. A *Celebration of Vegetables for Festive Meat-free Dining*. Macmillan, 1977.

Ahlquist, J.E.; Sibley, C.G. "Phylogeny of the Hominoid Primates as indicated by DNA-DNA Hybridization." *Journal of Molecular Evolution*, 20, 1984; pp 2–15.

American Heart Association. *1992 Heart and Stroke Facts Book*. AHA Books, 1992.

Anderson, J.W.; Spencer, D.B., et al. "Oat bran cereal lowers serum total and LDL cholesterol in hypercholesterolemic men." *American Journal of Clinical Nutrition*, 52, 1990; pp 495–499.

Baird, Pat. *Quick Harvest: A Vegetarian's Guide to Microwave Cooking*. Prentice-Hall, 1991.

Balboa, Deena; Balboa, David. *Walk for Life: The Lifetime Walking Program for a Healthy Body and Mind*. Penguin Books, 1990.

Barnard, Neal D., M.D. *The Power of Your Plate*. Book Publishing Company, 1990.

Benson, Herbert, M.D. *The Wellness Workbook*. Carol Publishing, 1992.

Berry, Ryan. *Famous Vegetarians and Their Recipes*. Panjandrum Books, 1990.

Black, Dean, Ph. D. *Health at the Crossroads*. Tapestry Press, 1988.

Borysenko, Joan, Ph. D. *Minding the Body, Mending the Mind*. Addison-Wesley, 1987.

Brenner, B.M., et al. "Dietary Protein Intake and the Progressive Nature of Kidney Disease." *New England Journal of Medicine*, 307, 1982; pp 652–659.

Burns, David M., M.D. *Feeling Good: The New Mood Therapy*. New American Library, 1981.

Chopra, Deepak, M.D. *Quantum Healing: Exploring the Frontiers of Bodymind Medicine*. Bantam, 1990.

Cooper, Kenneth H., M.D., M.P.H. *Aerobics Program for Total Wellbeing*. Bantam, 1988.; *Controlling Cholesterol Preventative Medicine Program*. Bantam, 1989.

Dahlberg, F., editor. *Woman the Gatherer*. Yale University Press, 1981.

Diamond, Jared (professor of physiology, UCLA School of Medicine). "Dawn of the Human Race." *Discover*, May 1989.

Diamond, Marilyn. *American Vegetarian Cookbook from the Fit For Life Kitchen*. (In production), 1992

Eaton S. Boyd., M.D.; Konner, Melvin J., M.D., Ph.D.; Shostak, Marjorie. "Stone Agers in the Fast Lane: Chronic and Degenerative Diseases in Evolutionary Perspective." *American Journal of Medicine*, 84, 1988; pp 735–747.; The Paleolithic Prescription, Harper & Row, 1989.

Ford, Norman D. *Good Health Without Drugs*. St. Martin's Press, 1979; *Natural Ways to Relieve Pain*. Harian Press, 1980; *Minding Your Body*. Autumn Press, 1981; *Arthritis and Gout*. Prentice Hall, 1982; *Good Night to*

Insomnia. Para Research, 1983; *Sleep Well, Live Well.* Zebra Books, 1984; *Lifestyle For Longevity.* Para Research, 1985; *Formula for Long Life.* Harian Press, 1985; *Eighteen Natural Ways to Beat the Common Cold.* Keats Publishing, 1987; *Eighteen Natural Ways to Beat a Headache.* Keats Publishing, 1988; *Keep on Pedaling.* Countryman Press, 1990; *The Healthiest Places to Live and Retire.* Ballantine Books, 1992; *Walk to Your Heart's Content.* Countryman Press, 1992.

Freeland-Graves, J. "Mineral Adequacy of Vegetarian Diets." *American Journal of Clinical Nutrition*, 48, 1988; pp 859–862.

Fuchs, Victor. *The Health Economy.* Harvard University Press, 1986.

Haberstroh, Chuck; Morris, Charles E. *Fat and Cholesterol Reduced Foods: Technologies and Strategies.* Portfolio Publications, 1991.

Hart, William. *Vipassana Meditation as Taught by S.N. Goenka.* Harper & Row, 1987.

Hittleman, Richard. *Richard Hittleman's 28-Day Yoga Exercise Plan.* Workman Publishing, 1969.

Inlander, Charles B.; Lowell, S. Levin. *Medicine on Trial.* Prentice-Hall, 1988.

Iyengar, B.K.S. *Light on Yoga.* Schocken Books, 1979.

Jampolsky, Gerald G., M.D. *Love is Letting Go of Fear.* Bantam 1981; *Goodbye to Guilt.* Bantam, 1985; *Out of Darkness into the Light.* Bantam, 1989.

Keyes, Ken. *Handbook to Higher Consciousness.* Love Line Books, 1975; *Handbook to Higher Consciousness: The Workbook.* Love Line Books, 1989.

Keys, Ancel. *Seven Countries: a Multivariate Analysis of Death and Coronary Disease.* Harvard University Press, 1980.

257

Krimmel, Patricia; Krimmel, Edward. *Cholesterol Lowering and Controlling*. Franklin Publishers, 1990.

Kushi, Aveline; Monte, Tom. *Thirty Days: Lower Cholesterol, Achieve Optimal Weight and Prevent Serious Disease*. Japan Publications, 1990.

Kwiterovich, Peter. *Beyond Cholesterol: Johns Hopkins Complete Guide for Avoiding Heart Disease*. Johns Hopkins, 1989; Knightsbridge Publications, 1991.

Lappé, Frances Moore. *Diet for a Small Planet*. Ballantine Books, 1982.

Larg, Susan S. "The World's Healthiest Diet (Chinese Diet Study)." *American Health*, September 1989; p. 105.

Leonard J.; Laut, P. *Rebirthing: The Science of Enjoying All of Your Life*. Trinity Press, 1983.

Lewis, Sylvan R. *Cholesterol Care Made Easy*. Lifetime Press, 1981.

Locke, Steven, M.D.; Colligan, Douglas. *The Healer Within*. New American Library, 1987.

McDougall, John, M.D. *The McDougall Plan*. New American Library–Dutton, 1991.

Maleskey, Gale. "Cure it With Walking—Seven Health Problems You Can Leave in the Dust." *Prevention*, September 1989; pp 90–128.

National Academy of Sciences. *Diet and Health: Implications for Reducing Chronic Disease Risk*. National Academy Press, 1989.

National Research Council. *Recommended Dietary Allowances*. National Academy Press, 1989.

Ornish, Dean. *Stress, Diet and Your Heart*. New American Library, Dutton, 1984; *Dr. Dean Ornish's Program for Reversing Heart Disease*. Random House, 1990; Ballantine Books, 1992.

Padus, Emrika. *Your Emotions and Your Health*. Rodale Press, 1986.

Paffenbarger, R.S. et al. "Physical Activity, All-Cause Mortality and Longevity of College Alumni." *New England Journal of Medicine*, 314, 1986; pp 605–613.

Pellet, P.L. "Protein Requirements in Humans." *American Journal of Clinical Nutrition*, 51, 1990; pp 723–737.

Perlmutter, Cathy. "Reverse Heart Disease Naturally." *Prevention*, May 1990: pp 50–60.

Pitchford, Paul. *Healing With Whole Foods*. North Atlantic Press, 1991.

Prevention Magazine's Editors. *Positive Living and Your Health*. Rodale Press, 1990.

Pritikin, Robert. *The New Pritikin Program* (includes recipes). Simon & Schuster, 1991.

Rachor, JoAnn. *Of These Ye May Freely Eat: A Vegetarian Cookbook*. Family Health Publishers, 1990.

Rippe, James M., M.D. *Dr. James M. Rippe's Complete Book of Fitness Walking*. Prentice-Hall, 1990.

Robertson, Laurel. *Laurel's Kitchen Bread Book*. Random House, 1985.

Robbins, John. *Diet for a New America*. Stillpoint Press, 1987.

Robbins, John; Mortiffe, Ann. *In Search of Balance: Discovering Harmony in a Changing World*. H. J. Kramer, 1991.

Satchidananda, Swami. *Integral Yoga Hatha*. Holt, Rinehart & Winston, 1970.

Schlossberg, Nancy, M.D. *Overwhelmed: Coping with Life's Ups and Downs*. Lexington Books, 1990.

Siegel, Bernie S., M.D., Ph. D. *Love, Medicine and Miracles*. HarperCollins, 1990; *Peace, Love and Healing: Bodymind Communications and the Path to Self-Healing*. HarperCollins, 1990.

Singer, Fred. *Change Your Mind, Save Your Life*. Colonial House Press, 1990.

Snowdon, D.A. et al. "Meat Consumption and Fatal Ischemic Heart Disease." *Preventive Medicine*, 1984.

Spilner, Maggie. "Seven Ways to Walk Away From Stress." *Prevention*, Jan.-Feb. 1991; pp 28–32.

U.S. Department of Human Health and Services. *Surgeon General's Report on Nutrition and Health*. Government Printing Office, 1988.

Vegetarian Times Editors. *Vegetarian Times Cookbook*. Macmillan, 1984.

Vishnudevananda, Swami. *The Complete Illustrated Book of Yoga*. Bell Publishing, 1960.

Wagner, Lindsay. *The High Road to Health* (recipes). Prentice-Hall, 1991.

Walford, Roy L., M.D. The 120-Year Diet. Archway, 1988.

Willet, W.C.; Stampfer, M.J. et al. "Relation of meat, fat and fiber intake to risk of colon cancer." *New England Journal of Medicine*, 323, 1990; pp 1664–1672.

Williams, Redford, M.D. *The Trusting Heart: Great News About Type A Behavior*. Random House, 1989.

Woods, B.; Martin, L.; Andrews, P. *Major Topics in Primate and Human Evolution*. Cambridge University Press, 1986.

World Health Organization. *Diet, Nutrition and the Prevention of Chronic Disease*. Geneva, 1990.

Yanker, Gary D. *Walking Medicine: The Lifetime Guide to Preventative Therapeutic and Exercise Walking Programs*. McGraw-Hill, 1990.

Yeagle, Phillip L. *The Biology of Cholesterol*. CRC Press, 1988; *Understanding Your Cholesterol*. Academy Press, 1991.

INDEX

A

Albert Einstein College of Medicine, New York City, 81
Alzheimer's Disease, 81
American Cancer Society, 99
American College of Pathologists, 30
American College of Sports Medicine, 193
American Diet:
   average cholesterol content, 62
   average fat content, 19, 62
   comparison to Chinese diet, 14
   fat and cholesterol overload, 13
   linked to cancer, 81
   part of culture, 10, 21–22
   U.S. government guidelines for, 213
American Dietetic Association, 86
American Health Foundation, 99
American Heart Association (AHA), 18, 61–62, 109, 199, 207
   Prudent Diet, 9, 17
      Step One, 9, 53, 83
      Step Two, 9, 53, 84
   Stop Smoking Program, 99
American lifestyle:

cause of high cholesterol epidemic, 4, 48
complacency about changing, 6
American Lung Association, 99
Angina, 44, 75, 99
   pain disappears, 16, 20
   helping your doctor phase out drugs for, 51
Angioplasty, 8, 78
Anti-oxidants, 73, 124, 206–210
Atherectomy, 8, 78
Atherosclerosis, 17, 61, 74
   in young American males, 75
Aversion Therapy, 101–102

B

Baltimore Longitudinal Study, 208
Barrett-Connor, Elizabeth, Ph. D., 141
Belief reprogramming, 235–242
Berkman, Lisa F., Ph. D., 243
Beta blockers, 31
Beta carotene, 73, 207–208
Biofeedback, using, 229–232
Birth control pills, 31
Björntorp, Per, Doctor, 199
Blair, Steven N., P.E.D., 48

261

263

ABOUT THE AUTHOR

Norman D. Ford is a medical researcher, a self-help author and an expert in holistic therapies. He has written for *Prevention* and *Bestways* and other well-known health magazines and has lectured extensively to health groups and organizations. Ford has authored more than forty books in the fields of retirement, leisure and health. He practices what he preaches and his lifestyle is built around the Whole Person health practices described in this book. An avid hiker, bicyclist, swimmer and vegetarian, Ford lives in the Texas Hill Country. He is an accredited member of the American Medical Writers Association.